GLUTEN-FREE COOKBOOK

52 Delicious Healthy Diets and Tasty Gluten Free Weekly Recipes For Everyday Life.

DEANNA BURNS

Table of Contents

Introduction

Chapter 1 Weekly Meal Plan

Chapter 2 Breakfast Recipes

1. Quick Sausage Cornmeal Pancakes

2. Berry Crepes

3. Bacon and Cheese Frittata

4. Vegetable Frittata

5. Egg Muffins

6. Baked Avocado Egg Boats

7. Berry-Chia Yogurt Parfait

8. Lean and Green Smoothie

9. Hawaiian Smoothie Bowl

10. Chickpea Pancakes with maple Yogurt Topping and Berries

Chapter 3 Other Breakfast Recipes

11. Tropical Pineapple Green Smoothie

12. Fluffy Scrambled Eggs, Sausage, Spinach, and Mushroom Bowl

13. Chocolate Chip Banana Bread Loaf

14. Chocolate Chip Oatmeal Chia Seed Muffins

15. Blueberry Oatmeal Muffins

16. Peanut Butter and Chocolate Swirl Overnight Oats

17. Sun-Dried Tomato Basil Frittata Muffins

18. Acai Smoothie Bowl

19. Honey-Nut Granola

Chapter 4 Lunch Recipes

20. Mediterranean Lamb Casserole

21. Lamb and Potato Casserole

22. Pork and Mushroom Casserole

23. Pork Roast and Cabbage

24. Korean-Style Honeyed Chicken

25. Cheese and Beef Meatballs

26. Creamy Corn and Pork Bits

27. Squash Quinoa Casserole

28. Pinto Bean Sloppy Joe Mix

29. Turkey Stew with Green Chilies

30. Mushroom Tomato with Onion Gravy

31. Greek Chicken Salad

Chapter 5 Lunch Recipes

32. Turkey Quinoa Salad

33. Tuna and Green Bean Salad

34. Greek Chicken Casserole

35. Hunter Style Chicken

36. Chicken with Almonds and Prunes

37. Lemon Rosemary Chicken

Chapter 6 Dinner Recipes

    38.   Baja Fish Tacos

    39.   Classic Crab Cakes

    40.   Shrimp Bibimbap

    41.   Coconut-Crusted Shrimp

    42.   Steamed Mussels

Chapter 7 Other Dinner Recipes

    43.   Seared Sea Scallops

    44.   Chile Lime Cod

    45.   Pan-Seared Chicken Breast with Sautéed Zucchini

    46.   Moroccan Chicken Tagine

    47.   Mediterranean Chicken with Buckwheat

    48.   Chicken Moussaka

    49.   Chicken and Artichoke Rice

    50.   Easy Chicken Parmigiana

Chapter 8 Snacks Recipe

    51.   Basil and Minced Pork Fajita

    52.   Tortilla Pocket

    53.   Crispy Honey Chili Pork Tenderloins

    54.   Chicken and Potato Taco

    55.   Mexican Cheese Poblanos

    56.   Three Cheese Nachos

    57.   Butter Cajun Shrimps

58. Smokey Chili Lamb Bites

59. Jalapeno Yogurt Balls

60. Potato and Green Pea Cutlets

Chapter 9 Other Snack Recipes

61. Avocado Crust California Pizza

62. Cauliflower Crust Margarita Pizza

63. Sweet Potato-Crusted Pizza with Sun-Dried Tomato Pesto, Portobello, and Grilled Chicken

64. Flatbread

65. Garlic Butter Flatbread Sticks

66. Graham Crackers

67. Gluten-Free Crackers

Chapter 10 Extra Side Recipes

68. Cream of Chicken Soup

69. Caldo de Pollo

70. Potato-Broccoli Soup

71. Cream of Mushroom Soup

72. Strawberry-Cucumber Salad

73. Mason Jar Taco Salad

74. Lemony Kale Salad with Parmesan and Golden Raisins

75. Easy Three-Bean Salad

76. Mustard Potato Salad

Conclusion

Introduction

A lot of people are turning gluten-free nowadays due to food allergies, intolerance or special food requirements, and if you are one of them, then it can be not easy to decide what to cook. It can prove to be helpful to have at least one gluten-free book on your bookshelf, for that friend who is suffering from celiac disease and is visiting you for some tea and snacks, or a bunch of vegetarians are coming over for lunch.

Gluten is a protein found in some grains. The two main proteins in gluten are gliadin and glutenin. When they come in contact with water, these proteins link and become gluten strands that build a web-like network, this substance becomes the "glue" that holds foods together and gives it stretch, elasticity, and beloved texture. This protein is found in grains such as wheat (including durum, semolina, kamut cereal, spelt, einkorn, triticale, and farro), barley, rye, and oats (unless the oats are certified gluten-free).

Gluten-related disorders are adverse reactions to the gluten protein. The level of sensitivity can range from a mild intolerance, which does not involve any antibodies, to celiac disease, in which the immune system attacks itself in response to eating gluten and prevents the body from properly absorbing food. Symptoms include bloating, diarrhea, infertility, osteoporosis, anemia, malnutrition, and neurological disorders, to name a few.

Gluten was initially being used back in the early 20th century as a food stabilizer, giving treats such as ice cream the density needed to prevent melting when handled by a customer. Today, it is used in most baked goods such as bread, pasta, crackers, muffins, pies, cakes, and pastries. Even unsuspecting items—soy sauce, salad dressing, soup, candy, toothpaste, shampoo, cleaning products, supplements, food coloring, Play-Doh, and beauty products—can ambush the unaware person with doses of gluten—isn't that crazy?

Gluten is present in an end number of foods; hence it can be challenging for so many people. Whether you want to remove gluten out of your meals or you are just cooking a meal for your friends or family with celiac disease, this recipe book will give you the tools which you require to gain encouragement and decide what to cook for a meal.

Flourishing gluten-free recipes need something more than new ingredients. You need to have a new system, and that's where this book can help you with. In this innovative recipe book, you will learn how to you can successfully cook many dishes without using wheat flour. And there is a reinvention of the system of baking to make delicious pies, cakes, casseroles, muffins and more.

It becomes rather difficult to switch to this beneficial diet as one may find themselves giving up a lot of the delicious food items. Well, initially every little endeavor takes a massive load on one's chest. Still, slowly over time if proper resources are available and one is determined enough, the transformation becomes much more manageable.

This wide-ranging recipe book will prove to be extremely helpful if you are preparing food for people with gluten intolerance or allergies. It consists of an extensive collection of recipes which are free from gluten.

Chapter 1 Weekly Meal Plan

WEEK 1

DAY	BREAKFAST	LUNCH	DINNER	SNACK
Monday	Quick Sausage Cornmeal Pancakes	Mediterranean Lamb Casserole	Baja Fish Tacos	Basil and Minced Pork Fajita
Tuesday	Quick Sausage Cornmeal Pancakes	Lamb And Potato Casserole	Classic Crab Cakes	Tortilla Pocket
Wednesday	Quick Sausage Cornmeal Pancakes	Pork and Mushroom Casserole	Shrimp Bibimbap	Crispy Honey Chili Pork Tenderloins
Thursday	Quick Sausage Cornmeal Pancakes	Pork Roast and Cabbage	Coconut-Crusted Shrimp	Chicken and Potato Taco

Friday	Quick Sausage Cornmeal Pancakes	Korean-Style Honeyed Chicken	Steamed Mussels	Mexican Cheese Poblanos
Saturday	Quick Sausage Cornmeal Pancakes	Creamy Corn and Pork Bits	Classic Crab Cakes	Tortilla Pocket
Sunday	Quick Sausage Cornmeal Pancakes	Pork Roast Cabbage	Chile Lime Cod	Chicken Potato Taco

WEEK 2

DAY	BREAKFAST	LUNCH	DINNER	SNACK
Monday	Berry Crepes	Cheese and Beef Meatballs	New England Clam Chowder	Three Cheese Nachos
Tuesday	Berry Crepes	Cheese and Beef Meatballs	Seared Sea Scallops	Butter Cajun Shrimps
Wednesday	Bacon And Cheese Frittata	Cheese and Beef Meatballs	Chile Lime Cod	Smokey Chili Lamb Bites
Thursday	Vegetable Frittata	Cheese and Beef Meatballs	Pan-Seared Chicken Breast with Sautéed Zucchini	Jalapeno Yogurt Balls
Friday	Egg Muffins	Cheese and Beef Meatballs	Moroccan Chicken Tagine	Potato and Green

				Pea Cutlet
Saturday	Honey-Nut Granola	Cheese and Beef Meatballs	Shrimp Bibimbap	Three Cheese Nachos
Sunday	Blueberry Oatmeal Muffins	Cheese and Beef Meatballs	Steamed Mussels	Jalapeno Yogurt Balls

WEEK 3

DAY	BREAKFAST	LUNCH	DINNER	SNACK
Monday	Baked Avocado Egg Boats	Creamy Corn and Pork Bits	Mediterranean Chicken with Buckwheat	Avocado Crust California Pizza
Tuesday	Berry-Chia Yogurt Parfait	Squash Quinoa Casserole	Mediterranean Chicken with Buckwheat	Cauliflower Crust Margarita Pizza
Wednesday	Lean And Green Smoothie	Pinto Bean Sloppy Joe Mix	Mediterranean Chicken with Buckwheat	Sweet Potato-Crusted Pizza with Sun-Dried Tomato Pesto, Portobello, and Grilled Chicken

Thursday	Hawaiian Smoothie Bowl	Turkey Stew with Green Chilies	Mediterranean Chicken with Buckwheat	Flatbread
Friday	Berry-Chia Yogurt Parfait	Mushroom Tomato with Onion Gravy	Mediterranean Chicken with Buckwheat	Garlic Butter Flatbread Sticks
Saturday	Egg Muffins	Pork and Mushroom Casserole	Mediterranean Chicken with Buckwheat	Tortilla Pocket
Sunday	Vegetable Frittata	Creamy Corn and Pork Bits	Mediterranean Chicken with Buckwheat	Chicken and Potato Taco

WEEK 4

DAY	BREAKFAST	LUNCH	DINNER	SNACK
Monday	Chickpea Pancakes With Maple Yogurt Topping And Berries	Greek Chicken Salad	Chicken Moussaka	Graham Crackers
Tuesday	Tropical Pineapple Green Smoothie	Turkey Quinoa Salad	Chicken and Artichoke Rice	Graham Crackers
Wednesday	Fluffy Scrambled Eggs	Tuna and Green Bean Salad	Easy Chicken Parmigiana	Graham Crackers
Thursday	Chocolate Chip Banana Bread Loaf	Greek Chicken Casserole	New England Clam Chowder	Graham Crackers

Friday	Chocolate Chip Oatmeal Chia Seed Muffins	Hunter Style Chicken	Seared Sea Scallops	Graham Crackers
Saturday	Quick Sausage Cornmeal Pancakes	Greek Chicken Salad	Chicken and Artichoke Rice	Graham Crackers
Sunday	Bacon and Cheese Frittata	Turkey Quinoa Salad	Easy Chicken Parmigiana	Graham Crackers

WEEK 5

DAY	BREAKFAST	LUNCH	DINNER	SNACK
Monday	Blueberry Oatmeal Muffins	Chicken with Almonds and Prunes	Chicken and Artichoke Rice	Gluten-Free Crackers
Tuesday	Blueberry Oatmeal Muffins	Lemon Rosemary Chicken	Chicken and Artichoke Rice	Three Cheese Nachos
Wednesday	Blueberry Oatmeal Muffins	Mediterranean Lamb Casserole	Chicken and Artichoke Rice	Butter Cajun Shrimps
Thursday	Blueberry Oatmeal Muffins	Lamb And Potato Casserole	Chicken and Artichoke Rice	Smokey Chili Lamb Bites

Friday	Blueberry Oatmeal Muffins	Pork and Mushroom Casserole	Chicken and Artichoke Rice	Jalapeno Yogurt Balls
Saturday	Vegetable Frittata	Lemon Rosemary Chicken	Chicken and Artichoke Rice	Gluten-Free Crackers
Sunday	Egg Muffins	Mediterranean Lamb Casserole	Chicken and Artichoke Rice	Three Cheese Nachos

WEEK 6

DAY	BREAKFAST	LUNCH	DINNER	SNACK
Monday	Peanut Butter and Chocolate Swirl Overnight Oats	Pinto Bean Sloppy Joe Mix	Shrimp Bibimbap	Smokey Chili Lamb Bites
Tuesday	Sun-Dried Tomato Basil Frittata Muffins	Turkey Stew with Green Chilies	Shrimp Bibimbap	Avocado Crust California Pizza
Wednesday	Acai Smoothie Bowl	Mushroom Tomato with Onion Gravy	Shrimp Bibimbap	Cauliflower Crust Margarita Pizza
Thursday	Honey-Nut Granola	Cheese and Beef Meatballs	Shrimp Bibimbap	Sweet Potato-Crusted Pizza with

20

				Sun-Dried Tomato Pesto, Portobello, and Grilled Chicken
Friday	Chickpea Pancakes With Maple Yogurt Topping And Berries	Cheese and Beef Meatballs	Shrimp Bibimbap	Flatbread
Saturday	Baked Avocado Egg Boats	Mushroom Tomato with Onion Gravy	Shrimp Bibimbap	Avocado Crust California Pizza
Sunday	Berry-Chia Yogurt Parfait	Cheese and Beef Meatballs	Shrimp Bibimbap	Cauliflower Crust Margarita Pizza

WEEK 7

DAY	BREAKFAST	LUNCH	DINNER	SNACK
Monday	Baked Avocado Egg Boats	Mushroom Tomato with Onion Gravy	Chicken Moussaka	Sweet Potato-Crusted Pizza with Sun-Dried Tomato Pesto, Portobello, and Grilled Chicken
Tuesday	Berry-Chia Yogurt Parfait	Cheese and Beef Meatballs	Chicken and Artichoke Rice	Flatbread
Wednesday	Lean And Green Smoothie	Cheese and Beef Meatballs	Easy Chicken Parmigiana	Garlic Butter

				Flatbread Sticks
Thursday	Hawaiian Smoothie Bowl	Korean-Style Honeyed Chicken	Mediterrane an Chicken with Buckwheat	Graham Cracker
Friday	Berry-Chia Yogurt Parfait	Pork and Mushroo m Casserole	Mediterrane an Chicken with Buckwheat	Jalapeno Yogurt Balls
Saturday	Lean and Green Smoothie	Korean-Style Honeyed Chicken	Mediterrane an Chicken with Buckwheat	Flatbread
Sunday	Hawaiian Smoothie Bowl	Pork and Mushroo m Casserole	Mediterrane an Chicken with Buckwheat	Garlic Butter Flatbread Sticks

WEEK 8

DAY	BREAKFAST	LUNCH	DINNER	SNACK
Monday	Quick Sausage Cornmeal Pancakes	Pork and Mushroom Casserole	Classic Crab Cakes	Cauliflower Crust Margarita Pizza
Tuesday	Berry Crepes	Pork Roast and Cabbage	Shrimp Bibimbap	Cauliflower Crust Margarita Pizza
Wednesday	Bacon And Cheese Frittata	Korean-Style Honeyed Chicken	Mediterranean Chicken with Buckwheat	Cauliflower Crust Margarita Pizza
Thursday	Vegetable Frittata	Pinto Bean Sloppy Joe Mix	Mediterranean Chicken with Buckwheat	Cauliflower Crust Margarita Pizza
Friday	Lean And Green Smoothie	Turkey Stew with Green Chilies	Chicken and Artichoke Rice	Cauliflower Crust Margarita Pizza

Saturday	Chickpea Pancakes with maple Yogurt Topping and Berries	Pork Roast and Cabbage	Classic Crab Cakes	Cauliflower Crust Margarita Pizza
Sunday	Tropical Pineapple Green Smoothie	Korean-Style Honeyed Chicken	Shrimp Bibimbap	Cauliflower Crust Margarita Pizza

WEEK 9

DAY	BREAKFAST	LUNCH	DINNER	SNACK
Monday	Acai Smoothie Bowl	Mediterranean Lamb Casserole	Baja Fish Tacos	Basil and Minced Pork Fajita

Tuesday	Honey-Nut Granola	Lamb And Potato Casserole	Classic Crab Cakes	Tortilla Pocket
Wednesday	Acai Smoothie Bowl	Pork and Mushroom Casserole	Shrimp Bibimbap	Crispy Honey Chili Pork Tenderloins
Thursday	Honey-Nut Granola	Pork Roast and Cabbage	Coconut-Crusted Shrimp	Chicken and Potato Taco
Friday	Honey-Nut Granola	Korean-Style Honeyed Chicken	Steamed Mussels	Mexican Cheese Poblanos
Saturday	Fluffy Scrambled Eggs, Sausage, Spinach, and Mushroom Bowl	Lamb And Potato Casserole	Classic Crab Cakes	Tortilla Pocket

| Sunday | Chocolate Chip Banana Bread Loaf | Pork and Mushroom Casserole | Shrimp Bibimbap | Crispy Honey Chili Pork Tenderloins |

WEEK 10

DAY	BREAKFAST	LUNCH	DINNER	SNACK
Monday	Baked Avocado Egg Boats	Creamy Corn and Pork Bits	Mediterranean Chicken with Buckwheat	Avocado Crust California Pizza
Tuesday	Berry-Chia Yogurt Parfait	Squash Quinoa Casserole	Mediterranean Chicken	Cauliflower Crust

			with Buckwheat	Margarita Pizza
Wednesday	Lean And Green Smoothie	Pinto Bean Sloppy Joe Mix	Mediterranean Chicken with Buckwheat	Sweet Potato-Crusted Pizza with Sun-Dried Tomato Pesto, Portobello, and Grilled Chicken
Thursday	Hawaiian Smoothie Bowl	Turkey Stew with Green Chilies	Mediterranean Chicken with Buckwheat	Flatbread
Friday	Berry-Chia Yogurt Parfait	Mushroom Tomato with Onion Gravy	Mediterranean Chicken with Buckwheat	Garlic Butter Flatbread Sticks

Saturday	Chocolate Chip Oatmeal Chia Seed Muffins	Pinto Bean Sloppy Joe Mix	Mediterranean Chicken with Buckwheat	Cauliflower Crust Margarita Pizza
Sunday	Blueberry Oatmeal Muffins	Turkey Stew with Green Chilies	Mediterranean Chicken with Buckwheat	Sweet Potato-Crusted Pizza with Sun-Dried Tomato Pesto, Portobello, and Grilled Chicken

WEEK 11

DAY	BREAKFAST	LUNCH	DINNER	SNACK
Monday	Berry Crepes	Cheese and Beef Meatballs	New England Clam Chowder	Three Cheese Nachos
Tuesday	Berry Crepes	Cheese and Beef Meatballs	Seared Sea Scallops	Butter Cajun Shrimps
Wednesday	Bacon And Cheese Frittata	Cheese and Beef Meatballs	Chile Lime Cod	Smokey Chili Lamb Bites
Thursday	Vegetable Frittata	Cheese and Beef Meatballs	Pan-Seared Chicken Breast with Sautéed Zucchini	Jalapeno Yogurt Balls
Friday	Egg Muffins	Cheese and Beef Meatballs	Moroccan Chicken Tagine	Potato and Green

				Pea Cutlet
Saturday	Peanut Butter and Chocolate Swirl Overnight Oats	Cheese and Beef Meatballs	New England Clam Chowder	Smokey Chili Lamb Bites
Sunday	Sun-Dried Tomato Basil Frittata Muffins	Cheese and Beef Meatballs	Seared Sea Scallops	Jalapeno Yogurt Balls

WEEK 12

DAY	BREAKFAST	LUNCH	DINNER	SNACK
Monday	Blueberry Oatmeal Muffins	Chicken with Almonds and Prunes	Chicken and Artichoke Rice	Gluten-Free Crackers
Tuesday	Blueberry Oatmeal Muffins	Lemon Rosemary Chicken	Chicken and Artichoke Rice	Three Cheese Nachos
Wednesday	Blueberry Oatmeal Muffins	Mediterranean Lamb Casserole	Chicken and Artichoke Rice	Butter Cajun Shrimps
Thursday	Blueberry Oatmeal Muffins	Lamb And Potato Casserole	Chicken and Artichoke Rice	Smokey Chili Lamb Bites
Friday	Blueberry Oatmeal Muffins	Pork and Mushroom Casserole	Chicken and Artichoke Rice	Jalapeno Yogurt Balls

| Saturday | Acai Smoothie Bowl | Lemon Rosemary Chicken | Chicken and Artichoke Rice | Three Cheese Nachos |
| Sunday | Honey-Nut Granola | Mediterranean Lamb Casserole | Chicken and Artichoke Rice | Butter Cajun Shrimps |

WEEK 13

DAY	BREAKFAST	LUNCH	DINNER	SNACK
Monday	Berry Crepes	Cheese and Beef Meatballs	New England	Three Cheese Nachos

			Clam Chowder	
Tuesday	Berry Crepes	Cheese and Beef Meatballs	Seared Sea Scallops	Butter Cajun Shrimps
Wednesday	Bacon And Cheese Frittata	Cheese and Beef Meatballs	Chile Lime Cod	Smokey Chili Lamb Bites
Thursday	Vegetable Frittata	Cheese and Beef Meatballs	Pan-Seared Chicken Breast with Sautéed Zucchini	Jalapeno Yogurt Balls
Friday	Egg Muffins	Cheese and Beef Meatballs	Moroccan Chicken Tagine	Potato and Green Pea Cutlet

Saturday	Quick Sausage Cornmeal Pancakes	Cheese and Beef Meatballs	Seared Sea Scallops	Butter Cajun Shrimps
Sunday	Berry Crepes	Cheese and Beef Meatballs	Chile Lime Cod	Smokey Chili Lamb Bites

WEEK 14

Monday	Acai Smoothie Bowl	Mediterranean Lamb Casserole	Baja Fish Tacos	Basil and Minced Pork Fajita

Tuesday	Honey-Nut Granola	Lamb And Potato Casserole	Classic Crab Cakes	Tortilla Pocket
Wednesday	Acai Smoothie Bowl	Pork and Mushroom Casserole	Shrimp Bibimbap	Crispy Honey Chili Pork Tenderloins
Thursday	Honey-Nut Granola	Pork Roast and Cabbage	Coconut-Crusted Shrimp	Chicken and Potato Taco
Friday	Honey-Nut Granola	Korean-Style Honeyed Chicken	Steamed Mussels	Mexican Cheese Poblanos
Monday	Acai Smoothie Bowl	Mediterranean Lamb Casserole	Baja Fish Tacos	Basil and Minced Pork Fajita
Saturday	Bacon and Cheese Frittata	Lamb And Potato Casserole	Baja Fish Tacos	Tortilla Pocket

Sunday	Vegetable Frittata	Pork and Mushroom Casserole	Classic Crab Cakes	Crispy Honey Chili Pork Tenderloins

WEEK 15

DAY	BREAKFAST	LUNCH	DINNER	SNACK
Monday	Baked Avocado Egg Boats	Creamy Corn and Pork Bits	Mediterranean Chicken with Buckwheat	Avocado Crust California Pizza

Tuesday	Berry-Chia Yogurt Parfait	Squash Quinoa Casserole	Mediterrane an Chicken with Buckwheat	Cauliflow er Crust Margarita Pizza
Wednesd ay	Lean And Green Smoothie	Pinto Bean Sloppy Joe Mix	Mediterrane an Chicken with Buckwheat	Sweet Potato- Crusted Pizza with Sun- Dried Tomato Pesto, Portobell o, and Grilled Chicken
Thursday	Hawaiian Smoothie Bowl	Turkey Stew with Green Chilies	Mediterrane an Chicken with Buckwheat	Flatbread
Friday	Berry-Chia Yogurt Parfait	Mushroo m Tomato with	Mediterrane an Chicken with Buckwheat	Garlic Butter Flatbread Sticks

		Onion Gravy		
Saturday	Egg Muffins	Pinto Bean Sloppy Joe Mix	Mediterrane an Chicken with Buckwheat	Sweet Potato-Crusted Pizza with Sun-Dried Tomato Pesto, Portobell o, and Grilled Chicken
Sunday	Baked Avocado Egg Boats	Turkey Stew with Green Chilies	Mediterrane an Chicken with Buckwheat	Flatbread

WEEK 16

DAY	BREAKFAST	LUNCH	DINNER	SNACK

Monday	Berry Crepes	Cheese and Beef Meatballs	New England Clam Chowder	Three Cheese Nachos
Tuesday	Berry Crepes	Cheese and Beef Meatballs	Seared Sea Scallops	Butter Cajun Shrimps
Wednesday	Bacon And Cheese Frittata	Cheese and Beef Meatballs	Chile Lime Cod	Smokey Chili Lamb Bites
Thursday	Vegetable Frittata	Cheese and Beef Meatballs	Pan-Seared Chicken Breast with Sautéed Zucchini	Jalapeno Yogurt Balls
Friday	Egg Muffins	Cheese and Beef Meatballs	Moroccan Chicken Tagine	Potato and Green Pea Cutlet

| Saturday | Berry-Chia Yogurt Parfait | Cheese and Beef Meatballs | New England Clam Chowder | Three Cheese Nachos |
| Sunday | Lean and Green Smoothie | Cheese and Beef Meatballs | Seared Sea Scallops | Butter Cajun Shrimps |

WEEK 17

DAY	BREAKFAST	LUNCH	DINNER	SNACK

Monday	Berry Crepes	Cheese and Beef Meatballs	New England Clam Chowder	Three Cheese Nachos
Tuesday	Berry Crepes	Cheese and Beef Meatballs	Seared Sea Scallops	Butter Cajun Shrimps
Wednesday	Bacon And Cheese Frittata	Cheese and Beef Meatballs	Chile Lime Cod	Smokey Chili Lamb Bites
Thursday	Vegetable Frittata	Cheese and Beef Meatballs	Pan-Seared Chicken Breast with Sautéed Zucchini	Jalapeno Yogurt Balls
Friday	Egg Muffins	Cheese and Beef Meatballs	Moroccan Chicken Tagine	Potato and Green Pea Cutlet

| Saturday | Hawaiian Smoothie Bowl | Cheese and Beef Meatballs | Seared Sea Scallops | Smokey Chili Lamb Bites |
| Sunday | Chickpea Pancakes with maple Yogurt Topping and Berries | Cheese and Beef Meatballs | Chile Lime Cod | Jalapeno Yogurt Balls |

WEEK 18

DAY	BREAKFAST	LUNCH	DINNER	SNACK

Monday	Acai Smoothie Bowl	Mediterranean Lamb Casserole	Baja Fish Tacos	Basil and Minced Pork Fajita
Tuesday	Honey-Nut Granola	Lamb And Potato Casserole	Classic Crab Cakes	Tortilla Pocket
Wednesday	Acai Smoothie Bowl	Pork and Mushroom Casserole	Shrimp Bibimbap	Crispy Honey Chili Pork Tenderloins
Thursday	Honey-Nut Granola	Pork Roast and Cabbage	Coconut-Crusted Shrimp	Chicken and Potato Taco
Friday	Honey-Nut Granola	Korean-Style Honeyed Chicken	Steamed Mussels	Mexican Cheese Poblanos
Saturday	Tropical Pineapple	Mediterranean Lamb	Classic Crab Cakes	Tortilla Pocket

	Green Smoothie	Casserole		
Sunday	Fluffy Scrambled Eggs, Sausage, Spinach, and Mushroom Bowl	Lamb And Potato Casserole	Shrimp Bibimbap	Crispy Honey Chili Pork Tenderloins

WEEK 19

DAY	BREAKFAST	LUNCH	DINNER	SNACK
Monday	Quick Sausage	Pork and Mushroo	Classic Crab Cakes	Cauliflower Crust

	Cornmeal Pancakes	m Casserole		Margarita Pizza
Tuesday	Berry Crepes	Pork Roast and Cabbage	Shrimp Bibimbap	Cauliflower Crust Margarita Pizza
Wednesday	Bacon And Cheese Frittata	Korean-Style Honeyed Chicken	Mediterranean Chicken with Buckwheat	Cauliflower Crust Margarita Pizza
Thursday	Vegetable Frittata	Pinto Bean Sloppy Joe Mix	Mediterranean Chicken with Buckwheat	Cauliflower Crust Margarita Pizza
Friday	Lean And Green Smoothie	Turkey Stew with Green Chilies	Chicken and Artichoke Rice	Cauliflower Crust Margarita Pizza
Saturday	Chocolate Chip Banana Bread Loaf	Korean-Style Honeyed Chicken	Classic Crab Cakes	Cauliflower Crust Margarita Pizza

Sunday	Chocolate Chip Oatmeal Chia Seed Muffins	Pinto Bean Sloppy Joe Mix	Shrimp Bibimbap	Cauliflower Crust Margarita Pizza

WEEK 20

DAY	BREAKFAST	LUNCH	DINNER	SNACK
Monday	Baked Avocado Egg Boats	Creamy Corn and Pork Bits	Mediterranean Chicken with Buckwheat	Avocado Crust California Pizza
Tuesday	Berry-Chia Yogurt Parfait	Squash Quinoa Casserole	Mediterranean Chicken with Buckwheat	Cauliflower Crust Margarita Pizza
Wednesday	Lean And Green Smoothie	Pinto Bean Sloppy Joe Mix	Mediterranean Chicken with Buckwheat	Sweet Potato-Crusted Pizza with Sun-Dried Tomato Pesto, Portobello, and Grilled Chicken

Thursday	Hawaiian Smoothie Bowl	Turkey Stew with Green Chilies	Mediterranean Chicken with Buckwheat	Flatbread
Friday	Berry-Chia Yogurt Parfait	Mushroom Tomato with Onion Gravy	Mediterranean Chicken with Buckwheat	Garlic Butter Flatbread Sticks
Saturday	Blueberry Oatmeal Muffins	Squash Quinoa Casserole	Mediterranean Chicken with Buckwheat	Avocado Crust California Pizza
Sunday	Peanut Butter and Chocolate Swirl Overnight Oats	Pinto Bean Sloppy Joe Mix	Mediterranean Chicken with Buckwheat	Cauliflower Crust Margarita Pizza

WEEK 21

DAY	BREAKFAST	LUNCH	DINNER	SNACK
Monday	Quick Sausage Cornmeal Pancakes	Pork and Mushroom Casserole	Classic Crab Cakes	Cauliflower Crust Margarita Pizza
Tuesday	Berry Crepes	Pork Roast and Cabbage	Shrimp Bibimbap	Cauliflower Crust Margarita Pizza
Wednesday	Bacon And Cheese Frittata	Korean-Style Honeyed Chicken	Mediterranean Chicken with Buckwheat	Cauliflower Crust Margarita Pizza
Thursday	Vegetable Frittata	Pinto Bean Sloppy Joe Mix	Mediterranean Chicken with Buckwheat	Cauliflower Crust Margarita Pizza
Friday	Lean And Green Smoothie	Turkey Stew with Green Chilies	Chicken and Artichoke Rice	Cauliflower Crust Margarita Pizza

Saturday	Sun-Dried Tomato Basil Frittata Muffins	Shrimp Bibimbap	Shrimp Bibimbap	Cauliflower Crust Margarita Pizza
Sunday	Acai Smoothie Bowl	Mediterranean Chicken with Buckwheat	Mediterranean Chicken with Buckwheat	Cauliflower Crust Margarita Pizza

WEEK 22

DAY	BREAKFAST	LUNCH	DINNER	SNACK
Monday	Acai Smoothie Bowl	Mediterranean Lamb Casserole	Baja Fish Tacos	Basil and Minced Pork Fajita
Tuesday	Honey-Nut Granola	Lamb And Potato Casserole	Classic Crab Cakes	Tortilla Pocket
Wednesday	Acai Smoothie Bowl	Pork and Mushroom Casserole	Shrimp Bibimbap	Crispy Honey Chili Pork Tenderloins
Thursday	Honey-Nut Granola	Pork Roast and Cabbage	Coconut-Crusted Shrimp	Chicken and Potato Taco
Friday	Honey-Nut Granola	Korean-Style Honeyed Chicken	Steamed Mussels	Mexican Cheese Poblanos

Saturday	Honey-Nut Granola	Pork Roast and Cabbage	Baja Fish Tacos	Basil and Minced Pork Fajita
Sunday	Acai Smoothie Bowl	Mediterranean Lamb Casserole	Coconut-Crusted Shrimp	Crispy Honey Chili Pork Tenderloins

WEEK 23

DAY	BREAKFAST	LUNCH	DINNER	SNACK
Monday	Baked Avocado Egg Boats	Creamy Corn and Pork Bits	Mediterranean Chicken with Buckwheat	Avocado Crust California Pizza
Tuesday	Berry-Chia Yogurt Parfait	Squash Quinoa Casserole	Mediterranean Chicken with Buckwheat	Cauliflower Crust Margarita Pizza
Wednesday	Lean And Green Smoothie	Pinto Bean Sloppy Joe Mix	Mediterranean Chicken with Buckwheat	Sweet Potato-Crusted Pizza with Sun-Dried Tomato Pesto, Portobello, and Grilled Chicken

Thursday	Hawaiian Smoothie Bowl	Turkey Stew with Green Chilies	Mediterranean Chicken with Buckwheat	Flatbread
Friday	Berry-Chia Yogurt Parfait	Mushroom Tomato with Onion Gravy	Mediterranean Chicken with Buckwheat	Garlic Butter Flatbread Sticks
Saturday	Lean And Green Smoothie	Turkey Stew with Green Chilies	Mediterranean Chicken with Buckwheat	Flatbread
Sunday	Baked Avocado Egg Boats	Squash Quinoa Casserole	Mediterranean Chicken with Buckwheat	Sweet Potato-Crusted Pizza with Sun-Dried Tomato Pesto, Portobello, and

				Grilled Chicken

WEEK 24

Monday	Acai Smoothie Bowl	Mediterranean Lamb Casserole	Baja Fish Tacos	Basil and Minced Pork Fajita
Tuesday	Honey-Nut Granola	Lamb And Potato Casserole	Classic Crab Cakes	Tortilla Pocket
Wednesday	Acai Smoothie Bowl	Pork and Mushroom Casserole	Shrimp Bibimbap	Crispy Honey Chili Pork Tenderloins
Thursday	Honey-Nut Granola	Pork Roast and Cabbage	Coconut-Crusted Shrimp	Chicken and Potato Taco
Friday	Honey-Nut Granola	Korean-Style Honeyed Chicken	Steamed Mussels	Mexican Cheese Poblanos
Monday	Acai Smoothie Bowl	Mediterranean Lamb Casserole	Baja Fish Tacos	Basil and Minced Pork Fajita

Saturday	Honey-Nut Granola	Lamb And Potato Casserole	Classic Crab Cakes	Tortilla Pocket
Sunday	Acai Smoothie Bowl	Pork Roast and Cabbage	Coconut-Crusted Shrimp	Crispy Honey Chili Pork Tenderloins

WEEK 25

DAY	BREAKFAST	LUNCH	DINNER	SNACK
Monday	Baked Avocado Egg Boats	Creamy Corn and Pork Bits	Mediterranean Chicken with Buckwheat	Avocado Crust California Pizza
Tuesday	Berry-Chia Yogurt Parfait	Squash Quinoa Casserole	Mediterranean Chicken with Buckwheat	Cauliflower Crust Margarita Pizza
Wednesday	Lean And Green Smoothie	Pinto Bean Sloppy Joe Mix	Mediterranean Chicken with Buckwheat	Sweet Potato-Crusted Pizza with Sun-Dried Tomato Pesto, Portobello, and Grilled Chicken

Thursday	Hawaiian Smoothie Bowl	Turkey Stew with Green Chilies	Mediterranean Chicken with Buckwheat	Flatbread
Friday	Berry-Chia Yogurt Parfait	Mushroom Tomato with Onion Gravy	Mediterranean Chicken with Buckwheat	Garlic Butter Flatbread Sticks
Saturday	Berry-Chia Yogurt Parfait	Creamy Corn and Pork Bits	Mediterranean Chicken with Buckwheat	Cauliflower Crust Margarita Pizza
Sunday	Baked Avocado Egg Boats	Pinto Bean Sloppy Joe Mix	Mediterranean Chicken with Buckwheat	Flatbread

WEEK 26

DAY	BREAKFAST	LUNCH	DINNER	SNACK
Monday	Quick Sausage Cornmeal Pancakes	Pork and Mushroom Casserole	Classic Crab Cakes	Cauliflower Crust Margarita Pizza
Tuesday	Berry Crepes	Pork Roast and Cabbage	Shrimp Bibimbap	Cauliflower Crust Margarita Pizza
Wednesday	Bacon And Cheese Frittata	Korean-Style Honeyed Chicken	Mediterranean Chicken with Buckwheat	Cauliflower Crust Margarita Pizza
Thursday	Vegetable Frittata	Pinto Bean Sloppy Joe Mix	Mediterranean Chicken with Buckwheat	Cauliflower Crust Margarita Pizza
Friday	Lean And Green Smoothie	Turkey Stew with Green Chilies	Chicken and Artichoke Rice	Cauliflower Crust Margarita Pizza

Saturday	Quick Sausage Cornmeal Pancakes	Pinto Bean Sloppy Joe Mix	Classic Crab Cakes	Cauliflower Crust Margarita Pizza
Sunday	Berry Crepes	Pork and Mushroom Casserole	Mediterranean Chicken with Buckwheat	Cauliflower Crust Margarita Pizza

WEEK 27

DAY	BREAKFAST	LUNCH	DINNER	SNACK
Monday	Berry Crepes	Cheese and Beef Meatballs	New England Clam Chowder	Three Cheese Nachos
Tuesday	Berry Crepes	Cheese and Beef Meatballs	Seared Sea Scallops	Butter Cajun Shrimps
Wednesday	Bacon And Cheese Frittata	Cheese and Beef Meatballs	Chile Lime Cod	Smokey Chili Lamb Bites
Thursday	Vegetable Frittata	Cheese and Beef Meatballs	Pan-Seared Chicken Breast with Sautéed Zucchini	Jalapeno Yogurt Balls
Friday	Egg Muffins	Cheese and Beef Meatballs	Moroccan Chicken Tagine	Potato and Green

				Pea Cutlet
Saturday	Egg Muffins	Cheese and Beef Meatballs	New England Clam Chowder	Three Cheese Nachos
Sunday	Bacon And Cheese Frittata	Cheese and Beef Meatballs	Chile Lime Cod	Smokey Chili Lamb Bites

WEEK 28

DAY	BREAKFAST	LUNCH	DINNER	SNACK
Monday	Berry Crepes	Cheese and Beef Meatballs	New England Clam Chowder	Three Cheese Nachos
Tuesday	Berry Crepes	Cheese and Beef Meatballs	Seared Sea Scallops	Butter Cajun Shrimps
Wednesday	Bacon And Cheese Frittata	Cheese and Beef Meatballs	Chile Lime Cod	Smokey Chili Lamb Bites
Thursday	Vegetable Frittata	Cheese and Beef Meatballs	Pan-Seared Chicken Breast with Sautéed Zucchini	Jalapeno Yogurt Balls
Friday	Egg Muffins	Cheese and Beef Meatballs	Moroccan Chicken Tagine	Potato and Green

				Pea Cutlet
Saturday	Berry Crepes	Cheese and Beef Meatballs	Pan-Seared Chicken Breast with Sautéed Zucchini	Butter Cajun Shrimps
Sunday	Bacon And Cheese Frittata	Cheese and Beef Meatballs	Seared Sea Scallops	Three Cheese Nachos

WEEK 29

DAY	BREAKFAST	LUNCH	DINNER	SNACK
Monday	Quick Sausage Cornmeal Pancakes	Mediterranean Lamb Casserole	Baja Fish Tacos	Basil and Minced Pork Fajita
Tuesday	Quick Sausage Cornmeal Pancakes	Lamb And Potato Casserole	Classic Crab Cakes	Tortilla Pocket
Wednesday	Quick Sausage Cornmeal Pancakes	Pork and Mushroom Casserole	Shrimp Bibimbap	Crispy Honey Chili Pork Tenderloins
Thursday	Quick Sausage Cornmeal Pancakes	Pork Roast and Cabbage	Coconut-Crusted Shrimp	Chicken and Potato Taco
Friday	Quick Sausage	Korean-Style	Steamed Mussels	Mexican Cheese Poblanos

	Cornmeal Pancakes	Honeyed Chicken		
Saturday	Quick Sausage Cornmeal Pancakes	Lamb And Potato Casserole	Classic Crab Cakes	Crispy Honey Chili Pork Tenderloins
Sunday	Quick Sausage Cornmeal Pancakes	Mediterranean Lamb Casserole	Baja Fish Tacos	Tortilla Pocket

WEEK 30

DAY	BREAKFAST	LUNCH	DINNER	SNACK
Monday	Berry Crepes	Cheese and Beef Meatballs	New England Clam Chowder	Three Cheese Nachos
Tuesday	Berry Crepes	Cheese and Beef Meatballs	Seared Sea Scallops	Butter Cajun Shrimps
Wednesday	Bacon And Cheese Frittata	Cheese and Beef Meatballs	Chile Lime Cod	Smokey Chili Lamb Bites
Thursday	Vegetable Frittata	Cheese and Beef Meatballs	Pan-Seared Chicken Breast with Sautéed Zucchini	Jalapeno Yogurt Balls
Friday	Egg Muffins	Cheese and Beef Meatballs	Moroccan Chicken Tagine	Potato and Green

				Pea Cutlet
Saturday	Vegetable Frittata	Cheese and Beef Meatballs	Seared Sea Scallops	Butter Cajun Shrimps
Sunday	Berry Crepes	Cheese and Beef Meatballs	New England Clam Chowder	Three Cheese Nachos

WEEK 31

DAY	BREAKFAST	LUNCH	DINNER	SNACK
Monday	Baked Avocado Egg Boats	Creamy Corn and Pork Bits	Mediterranean Chicken with Buckwheat	Avocado Crust California Pizza
Tuesday	Berry-Chia Yogurt Parfait	Squash Quinoa Casserole	Mediterranean Chicken with Buckwheat	Cauliflower Crust Margarita Pizza
Wednesday	Lean And Green Smoothie	Pinto Bean Sloppy Joe Mix	Mediterranean Chicken with Buckwheat	Sweet Potato-Crusted Pizza with Sun-Dried Tomato Pesto, Portobello, and Grilled Chicken

Thursday	Hawaiian Smoothie Bowl	Turkey Stew with Green Chilies	Mediterranean Chicken with Buckwheat	Flatbread
Friday	Berry-Chia Yogurt Parfait	Mushroom Tomato with Onion Gravy	Mediterranean Chicken with Buckwheat	Garlic Butter Flatbread Sticks
Saturday	Lean And Green Smoothie	Mushroom Tomato with Onion Gravy	Mediterranean Chicken with Buckwheat	Flatbread
Sunday	Baked Avocado Egg Boats	Mushroom Tomato with Onion Gravy	Mediterranean Chicken with Buckwheat	Sweet Potato-Crusted Pizza with Sun-Dried Tomato Pesto,

				Portobello, and Grilled Chicken

WEEK 32

DAY	BREAKFAST	LUNCH	DINNER	SNACK
Monday	Quick Sausage Cornmeal Pancakes	Pork and Mushroom Casserole	Classic Crab Cakes	Cauliflower Crust Margarita Pizza
Tuesday	Berry Crepes	Pork Roast and Cabbage	Shrimp Bibimbap	Cauliflower Crust Margarita Pizza
Wednesday	Bacon And Cheese Frittata	Korean-Style Honeyed Chicken	Mediterranean Chicken with Buckwheat	Cauliflower Crust Margarita Pizza
Thursday	Vegetable Frittata	Pinto Bean Sloppy Joe Mix	Mediterranean Chicken with Buckwheat	Cauliflower Crust Margarita Pizza
Friday	Lean And Green Smoothie	Turkey Stew with Green Chilies	Chicken and Artichoke Rice	Cauliflower Crust Margarita Pizza

Saturday	Bacon And Cheese Frittata	Turkey Stew with Green Chilies	Classic Crab Cakes	Cauliflower Crust Margarita Pizza
Sunday	Quick Sausage Cornmeal Pancakes	Pork Roast and Cabbage	Shrimp Bibimbap	Cauliflower Crust Margarita Pizza

WEEK 33

DAY	BREAKFAST	LUNCH	DINNER	SNACK
Monday	Baked Avocado Egg Boats	Creamy Corn and Pork Bits	Mediterranean Chicken with Buckwheat	Avocado Crust California Pizza
Tuesday	Berry-Chia Yogurt Parfait	Squash Quinoa Casserole	Mediterranean Chicken with Buckwheat	Cauliflower Crust Margarita Pizza
Wednesday	Lean And Green Smoothie	Pinto Bean Sloppy Joe Mix	Mediterranean Chicken with Buckwheat	Sweet Potato-Crusted Pizza with Sun-Dried Tomato Pesto, Portobello, and Grilled Chicken

Thursday	Hawaiian Smoothie Bowl	Turkey Stew with Green Chilies	Mediterranean Chicken with Buckwheat	Flatbread
Friday	Berry-Chia Yogurt Parfait	Mushroom Tomato with Onion Gravy	Mediterranean Chicken with Buckwheat	Garlic Butter Flatbread Sticks
Saturday	Baked Avocado Egg Boats	Pinto Bean Sloppy Joe Mix	Mediterranean Chicken with Buckwheat	Sweet Potato-Crusted Pizza with Sun-Dried Tomato Pesto, Portobello, and Grilled Chicken

Sunday	Hawaiian Smoothie Bowl	Creamy Corn and Pork Bits	Mediterranean Chicken with Buckwheat	Cauliflower Crust Margarita Pizza

WEEK 34

DAY	BREAKFAST	LUNCH	DINNER	SNACK
Monday	Baked Avocado Egg Boats	Creamy Corn and Pork Bits	Mediterranean Chicken with Buckwheat	Avocado Crust California Pizza
Tuesday	Berry-Chia Yogurt Parfait	Squash Quinoa Casserole	Mediterranean Chicken with Buckwheat	Cauliflower Crust Margarita Pizza
Wednesday	Lean And Green Smoothie	Pinto Bean Sloppy Joe Mix	Mediterranean Chicken with Buckwheat	Sweet Potato-Crusted Pizza with Sun-Dried Tomato Pesto, Portobello, and Grilled Chicken

Thursday	Hawaiian Smoothie Bowl	Turkey Stew with Green Chilies	Mediterranean Chicken with Buckwheat	Flatbread
Friday	Berry-Chia Yogurt Parfait	Mushroom Tomato with Onion Gravy	Mediterranean Chicken with Buckwheat	Garlic Butter Flatbread Sticks
Saturday	Lean And Green Smoothie	Pinto Bean Sloppy Joe Mix	Mediterranean Chicken with Buckwheat	Avocado Crust California Pizza
Sunday	Hawaiian Smoothie Bowl	Mushroom Tomato with Onion Gravy	Mediterranean Chicken with Buckwheat	Sweet Potato-Crusted Pizza with Sun-Dried Tomato Pesto, Portobello, and

				Grilled Chicken

WEEK 35

DAY	BREAKFAST	LUNCH	DINNER	SNACK
Monday	Quick Sausage Cornmeal Pancakes	Mediterranean Lamb Casserole	Baja Fish Tacos	Basil and Minced Pork Fajita
Tuesday	Quick Sausage Cornmeal Pancakes	Lamb And Potato Casserole	Classic Crab Cakes	Tortilla Pocket
Wednesday	Quick Sausage Cornmeal Pancakes	Pork and Mushroom Casserole	Shrimp Bibimbap	Crispy Honey Chili Pork Tenderloins
Thursday	Quick Sausage Cornmeal Pancakes	Pork Roast and Cabbage	Coconut-Crusted Shrimp	Chicken and Potato Taco
Friday	Quick Sausage	Korean-Style	Steamed Mussels	Mexican Cheese Poblanos

	Cornmeal Pancakes	Honeyed Chicken		
Saturday	Quick Sausage Cornmeal Pancakes	Pork Roast and Cabbage	Classic Crab Cakes	Crispy Honey Chili Pork Tenderloins
Sunday	Quick Sausage Cornmeal Pancakes	Lamb And Potato Casserole	Coconut -Crusted Shrimp	Tortilla Pocket

WEEK 36

DAY	BREAKFAST	LUNCH	DINNER	SNACK
Monday	Quick Sausage Cornmeal Pancakes	Mediterranean Lamb Casserole	Baja Fish Tacos	Basil and Minced Pork Fajita
Tuesday	Quick Sausage Cornmeal Pancakes	Lamb And Potato Casserole	Classic Crab Cakes	Tortilla Pocket
Wednesday	Quick Sausage Cornmeal Pancakes	Pork and Mushroom Casserole	Shrimp Bibimbap	Crispy Honey Chili Pork Tenderloins
Thursday	Quick Sausage Cornmeal Pancakes	Pork Roast and Cabbage	Coconut-Crusted Shrimp	Chicken and Potato Taco
Friday	Quick Sausage	Korean-Style	Steamed Mussels	Mexican Cheese Poblanos

	Cornmeal Pancakes	Honeyed Chicken		
Saturday	Quick Sausage Cornmeal Pancakes	Mediterrane an Lamb Casserole	Shrimp Bibimba p	Basil and Minced Pork Fajita
Sunday	Quick Sausage Cornmeal Pancakes	Lamb And Potato Casserole	Baja Fish Tacos	Mexican Cheese Poblanos

WEEK 37

DAY	BREAKFAST	LUNCH	DINNER	SNACK
Monday	Berry Crepes	Cheese and Beef Meatballs	New England	Three Cheese Nachos

			Clam Chowder	
Tuesday	Berry Crepes	Cheese and Beef Meatballs	Seared Sea Scallops	Butter Cajun Shrimps
Wednesday	Bacon And Cheese Frittata	Cheese and Beef Meatballs	Chile Lime Cod	Smokey Chili Lamb Bites
Thursday	Vegetable Frittata	Cheese and Beef Meatballs	Pan-Seared Chicken Breast with Sautéed Zucchini	Jalapeno Yogurt Balls
Friday	Egg Muffins	Cheese and Beef Meatballs	Moroccan Chicken Tagine	Potato and Green Pea Cutlet

Saturday	Bacon And Cheese Frittata	Cheese and Beef Meatballs	Chile Lime Cod	Three Cheese Nachos
Sunday	Vegetable Frittata	Cheese and Beef Meatballs	Moroccan Chicken Tagine	Smokey Chili Lamb Bites

WEEK 38

DAY	BREAKFAST	LUNCH	DINNER	SNACK
Monday	Quick Sausage Cornmeal Pancakes	Pork and Mushroom Casserole	Classic Crab Cakes	Cauliflower Crust Margarita Pizza
Tuesday	Berry Crepes	Pork Roast and Cabbage	Shrimp Bibimbap	Cauliflower Crust Margarita Pizza
Wednesday	Bacon And Cheese Frittata	Korean-Style Honeyed Chicken	Mediterranean Chicken with Buckwheat	Cauliflower Crust Margarita Pizza
Thursday	Vegetable Frittata	Pinto Bean Sloppy Joe Mix	Mediterranean Chicken with Buckwheat	Cauliflower Crust Margarita Pizza
Friday	Lean And Green Smoothie	Turkey Stew with Green Chilies	Chicken and Artichoke Rice	Cauliflower Crust Margarita Pizza

Saturday	Berry Crepes	Korean-Style Honeyed Chicken	Classic Crab Cakes	Cauliflower Crust Margarita Pizza
Sunday	Quick Sausage Cornmeal Pancakes	Turkey Stew with Green Chilies	Mediterranean Chicken with Buckwheat	Cauliflower Crust Margarita Pizza

WEEK 39

DAY	BREAKFAST	LUNCH	DINNER	SNACK
Monday	Acai Smoothie Bowl	Mediterranean Lamb Casserole	Baja Fish Tacos	Basil and Minced Pork Fajita
Tuesday	Honey-Nut Granola	Lamb And Potato Casserole	Classic Crab Cakes	Tortilla Pocket
Wednesday	Acai Smoothie Bowl	Pork and Mushroom Casserole	Shrimp Bibimbap	Crispy Honey Chili Pork Tenderloins
Thursday	Honey-Nut Granola	Pork Roast and Cabbage	Coconut-Crusted Shrimp	Chicken and Potato Taco
Friday	Honey-Nut Granola	Korean-Style Honeyed Chicken	Steamed Mussels	Mexican Cheese Poblanos

Saturday	Acai Smoothie Bowl	Pork and Mushroom Casserole	Classic Crab Cakes	Crispy Honey Chili Pork Tenderloins
Sunday	Honey-Nut Granola	Mediterranean Lamb Casserole	Shrimp Bibimbap	Mexican Cheese Poblanos

WEEK 40

DAY	BREAKFAST	LUNCH	DINNER	SNACK
Monday	Acai Smoothie Bowl	Mediterranean Lamb Casserole	Baja Fish Tacos	Basil and Minced Pork Fajita
Tuesday	Honey-Nut Granola	Lamb And Potato Casserole	Classic Crab Cakes	Tortilla Pocket
Wednesday	Acai Smoothie Bowl	Pork and Mushroom Casserole	Shrimp Bibimbap	Crispy Honey Chili Pork Tenderloins
Thursday	Honey-Nut Granola	Pork Roast and Cabbage	Coconut-Crusted Shrimp	Chicken and Potato Taco
Friday	Honey-Nut Granola	Korean-Style Honeyed Chicken	Steamed Mussels	Mexican Cheese Poblanos

Saturday	Acai Smoothie Bowl	Lamb And Potato Casserole	Shrimp Bibimbap	Basil and Minced Pork Fajita
Sunday	Honey-Nut Granola	Pork Roast and Cabbage	Baja Fish Tacos	Tortilla Pocket

WEEK 41

DAY	BREAKFAST	LUNCH	DINNER	SNACK
Monday	Berry Crepes	Cheese and Beef Meatballs	New England Clam Chowder	Three Cheese Nachos
Tuesday	Berry Crepes	Cheese and Beef Meatballs	Seared Sea Scallops	Butter Cajun Shrimps
Wednesday	Bacon And Cheese Frittata	Cheese and Beef Meatballs	Chile Lime Cod	Smokey Chili Lamb Bites
Thursday	Vegetable Frittata	Cheese and Beef Meatballs	Pan-Seared Chicken Breast with Sautéed Zucchini	Jalapeno Yogurt Balls
Friday	Egg Muffins	Cheese and Beef Meatballs	Moroccan Chicken Tagine	Potato and Green

				Pea Cutlet
Saturday	Berry Crepes	Cheese and Beef Meatballs	New England Clam Chowder	Smokey Chili Lamb Bites
Sunday	Vegetable Frittata	Cheese and Beef Meatballs	Pan-Seared Chicken Breast with Sautéed Zucchini	Three Cheese Nachos

WEEK 42

DAY	BREAKFAST	LUNCH	DINNER	SNACK
Monday	Baked Avocado Egg Boats	Creamy Corn and Pork Bits	Mediterranean Chicken with Buckwheat	Avocado Crust California Pizza
Tuesday	Berry-Chia Yogurt Parfait	Squash Quinoa Casserole	Mediterranean Chicken with Buckwheat	Cauliflower Crust Margarita Pizza
Wednesday	Lean And Green Smoothie	Pinto Bean Sloppy Joe Mix	Mediterranean Chicken with Buckwheat	Sweet Potato-Crusted Pizza with Sun-Dried Tomato Pesto, Portobello, and Grilled Chicken

Thursday	Hawaiian Smoothie Bowl	Turkey Stew with Green Chilies	Mediterranean Chicken with Buckwheat	Flatbread
Friday	Berry-Chia Yogurt Parfait	Mushroom Tomato with Onion Gravy	Mediterranean Chicken with Buckwheat	Garlic Butter Flatbread Sticks
Saturday	Hawaiian Smoothie Bowl	Squash Quinoa Casserole	Mediterranean Chicken with Buckwheat	Sweet Potato-Crusted Pizza with Sun-Dried Tomato Pesto, Portobello, and Grilled Chicken

Sunday	Baked Avocado Egg Boats	Pinto Bean Sloppy Joe Mix	Mediterranean Chicken with Buckwheat	Flatbread

WEEK 43

DAY	BREAKFAST	LUNCH	DINNER	SNACK
Monday	Acai Smoothie Bowl	Mediterranean Lamb Casserole	Baja Fish Tacos	Basil and Minced Pork Fajita
Tuesday	Honey-Nut Granola	Lamb And Potato Casserole	Classic Crab Cakes	Tortilla Pocket
Wednesday	Acai Smoothie Bowl	Pork and Mushroom Casserole	Shrimp Bibimbap	Crispy Honey Chili Pork Tenderloins
Thursday	Honey-Nut Granola	Pork Roast and Cabbage	Coconut-Crusted Shrimp	Chicken and Potato Taco
Friday	Honey-Nut Granola	Korean-Style	Steamed Mussels	Mexican Cheese Poblanos

		Honeyed Chicken		
Saturday	Acai Smoothie Bowl	Pork and Mushroom Casserole	Coconut -Crusted Shrimp	Basil and Minced Pork Fajita
Sunday	Honey-Nut Granola	Pork Roast and Cabbage	Steamed Mussels	Tortilla Pocket

WEEK 44

DAY	BREAKFAST	LUNCH	DINNER	SNACK
Monday	Baked Avocado Egg Boats	Creamy Corn and Pork Bits	Mediterranean Chicken with Buckwheat	Avocado Crust California Pizza
Tuesday	Berry-Chia Yogurt Parfait	Squash Quinoa Casserole	Mediterranean Chicken with Buckwheat	Cauliflower Crust Margarita Pizza
Wednesday	Lean And Green Smoothie	Pinto Bean Sloppy Joe Mix	Mediterranean Chicken with Buckwheat	Sweet Potato-Crusted Pizza with Sun-Dried Tomato Pesto, Portobello, and Grilled Chicken

Thursday	Hawaiian Smoothie Bowl	Turkey Stew with Green Chilies	Mediterrane an Chicken with Buckwheat	Flatbread
Friday	Berry-Chia Yogurt Parfait	Mushroo m Tomato with Onion Gravy	Mediterrane an Chicken with Buckwheat	Garlic Butter Flatbread Sticks
Saturday	Berry-Chia Yogurt Parfait	Squash Quinoa Casserole	Mediterrane an Chicken with Buckwheat	Cauliflow er Crust Margarita Pizza
Sunday	Lean And Green Smoothie	Pinto Bean Sloppy Joe Mix	Mediterrane an Chicken with Buckwheat	Sweet Potato- Crusted Pizza with Sun- Dried Tomato Pesto, Portobell o, and

				Grilled Chicken

WEEK 45

DAY	BREAKFAST	LUNCH	DINNER	SNACK
Monday	Baked Avocado Egg Boats	Creamy Corn and Pork Bits	Mediterranean Chicken with Buckwheat	Avocado Crust California Pizza
Tuesday	Berry-Chia Yogurt Parfait	Squash Quinoa Casserole	Mediterranean Chicken with Buckwheat	Cauliflower Crust Margarita Pizza
Wednesday	Lean And Green Smoothie	Pinto Bean Sloppy Joe Mix	Mediterranean Chicken with Buckwheat	Sweet Potato-Crusted Pizza with Sun-Dried Tomato Pesto, Portobello, and Grilled Chicken

Thursday	Hawaiian Smoothie Bowl	Turkey Stew with Green Chilies	Mediterranean Chicken with Buckwheat	Flatbread
Friday	Berry-Chia Yogurt Parfait	Mushroom Tomato with Onion Gravy	Mediterranean Chicken with Buckwheat	Garlic Butter Flatbread Sticks
Saturday	Baked Avocado Egg Boats	Pinto Bean Sloppy Joe Mix	Mediterranean Chicken with Buckwheat	Sweet Potato-Crusted Pizza with Sun-Dried Tomato Pesto, Portobello, and Grilled Chicken

Sunday	Berry-Chia Yogurt Parfait	Turkey Stew with Green Chilies	Mediterranean Chicken with Buckwheat	Flatbread

WEEK 46

DAY	BREAKFAST	LUNCH	DINNER	SNACK
Monday	Acai Smoothie Bowl	Mediterranean Lamb Casserole	Baja Fish Tacos	Basil and Minced Pork Fajita
Tuesday	Honey-Nut Granola	Lamb And Potato Casserole	Classic Crab Cakes	Tortilla Pocket
Wednesday	Acai Smoothie Bowl	Pork and Mushroom Casserole	Shrimp Bibimbap	Crispy Honey Chili Pork Tenderloins
Thursday	Honey-Nut Granola	Pork Roast and Cabbage	Coconut-Crusted Shrimp	Chicken and Potato Taco
Friday	Honey-Nut Granola	Korean-Style Honeyed Chicken	Steamed Mussels	Mexican Cheese Poblanos

Saturday	Acai Smoothie Bowl	Lamb And Potato Casserole	Baja Fish Tacos	Crispy Honey Chili Pork Tenderloins
Sunday	Honey-Nut Granola	Pork and Mushroom Casserole	Classic Crab Cakes	Chicken and Potato Taco

WEEK 47

DAY	BREAKFAST	LUNCH	DINNER	SNACK
Monday	Baked Avocado Egg Boats	Creamy Corn and Pork Bits	Mediterranean Chicken with Buckwheat	Avocado Crust California Pizza
Tuesday	Berry-Chia Yogurt Parfait	Squash Quinoa Casserole	Mediterranean Chicken with Buckwheat	Cauliflower Crust Margarita Pizza
Wednesday	Lean And Green Smoothie	Pinto Bean Sloppy Joe Mix	Mediterranean Chicken with Buckwheat	Sweet Potato-Crusted Pizza with Sun-Dried Tomato Pesto, Portobello, and Grilled Chicken

Thursday	Hawaiian Smoothie Bowl	Turkey Stew with Green Chilies	Mediterranean Chicken with Buckwheat	Flatbread
Friday	Berry-Chia Yogurt Parfait	Mushroom Tomato with Onion Gravy	Mediterranean Chicken with Buckwheat	Garlic Butter Flatbread Sticks
Saturday	Berry-Chia Yogurt Parfait	Squash Quinoa Casserole	Mediterranean Chicken with Buckwheat	Avocado Crust California Pizza
Sunday	Lean And Green Smoothie	Pinto Bean Sloppy Joe Mix	Mediterranean Chicken with Buckwheat	Cauliflower Crust Margarita Pizza

WEEK 48

DAY	BREAKFAST	LUNCH	DINNER	SNACK
Monday	Berry Crepes	Cheese and Beef Meatballs	New England Clam Chowder	Three Cheese Nachos
Tuesday	Berry Crepes	Cheese and Beef Meatballs	Seared Sea Scallops	Butter Cajun Shrimps
Wednesday	Bacon And Cheese Frittata	Cheese and Beef Meatballs	Chile Lime Cod	Smokey Chili Lamb Bites
Thursday	Vegetable Frittata	Cheese and Beef Meatballs	Pan-Seared Chicken Breast with Sautéed Zucchini	Jalapeno Yogurt Balls
Friday	Egg Muffins	Cheese and Beef Meatballs	Moroccan Chicken Tagine	Potato and Green

				Pea Cutlet
Saturday	Berry Crepes	Cheese and Beef Meatballs	New England Clam Chowder	Smokey Chili Lamb Bites
Sunday	Bacon And Cheese Frittata	Cheese and Beef Meatballs	Seared Sea Scallops	Jalapeno Yogurt Balls

WEEK 49

DAY	BREAKFAST	LUNCH	DINNER	SNACK
Monday	Quick Sausage Cornmeal Pancakes	Berry Crepes	Classic Crab Cakes	Cauliflower Crust Margarita Pizza
Tuesday	Berry Crepes	Bacon And Cheese Frittata	Shrimp Bibimbap	Cauliflower Crust Margarita Pizza
Wednesday	Bacon And Cheese Frittata	Korean-Style Honeyed Chicken	Mediterranean Chicken with Buckwheat	Cauliflower Crust Margarita Pizza
Thursday	Vegetable Frittata	Pinto Bean Sloppy Joe Mix	Mediterranean Chicken with Buckwheat	Cauliflower Crust Margarita Pizza
Friday	Lean And Green Smoothie	Turkey Stew with	Chicken and Artichoke Rice	Cauliflower Crust

		Green Chilies		Margarita Pizza
Saturday	Berry Crepes	Berry Crepes	Classic Crab Cakes	Cauliflower Crust Margarita Pizza
Sunday	Bacon And Cheese Frittata	Bacon And Cheese Frittata	Classic Crab Cakes	Cauliflower Crust Margarita Pizza

WEEK 50

DAY	BREAKFAST	LUNCH	DINNER	SNACK
Monday	Peanut Butter and Chocolate Swirl Overnight Oats	Pinto Bean Sloppy Joe Mix	Shrimp Bibimbap	Smokey Chili Lamb Bites
Tuesday	Sun-Dried Tomato Basil Frittata Muffins	Turkey Stew with Green Chilies	Shrimp Bibimbap	Avocado Crust California Pizza
Wednesday	Acai Smoothie Bowl	Mushroom Tomato with Onion Gravy	Shrimp Bibimbap	Cauliflower Crust Margarita Pizza
Thursday	Honey-Nut Granola	Cheese and Beef Meatballs	Shrimp Bibimbap	Sweet Potato-Crusted Pizza with

				Sun-Dried Tomato Pesto, Portobello, and Grilled Chicken
Friday	Chickpea Pancakes With Maple Yogurt Topping And Berries	Cheese and Beef Meatballs	Shrimp Bibimba p	Flatbread
Saturday	Sun-Dried Tomato Basil Frittata Muffins	Pinto Bean Sloppy Joe Mix	Shrimp Bibimba p	Avocado Crust California Pizza
Sunday	Acai Smoothie Bowl	Turkey Stew with Green Chilies	Shrimp Bibimba p	Cauliflowe r Crust Margarita Pizza

WEEK 51

DAY	BREAKFAST	LUNCH	DINNER	SNACK
Monday	Quick Sausage Cornmeal Pancakes	Mediterranean Lamb Casserole	Baja Fish Tacos	Crispy Honey Chili Pork Tenderloins
Tuesday	Berry Crepes	Lamb and Potato Casserole	Coconut-Crusted Shrimp	Crispy Honey Chili Pork Tenderloins
Wednesday	Vegetable Frittata	Cheese and Beef Meatballs	Steamed Mussels	Crispy Honey Chili Pork Tenderloins

Thursday	Egg Muffins	Pork and Mushroom Casserole	Seared Sea Scallops	Crispy Honey Chili Pork Tenderloins
Friday	Baked Avocado Egg Boats	Pork Roast and Cabbage	Chile Lime Cod	Crispy Honey Chili Pork Tenderloins
Saturday	Berry-Chia Yogurt Parfait	Mediterranean Lamb Casserole	Pan-Seared Chicken Breast with Sautéed Zucchini	Crispy Honey Chili Pork Tenderloins
Sunday	Hawaiian Smoothie Bowl	Lamb and Potato Casserole	Mediterranean Chicken with Buckwheat	Crispy Honey Chili Pork Tenderloins

WEEK 52

DAY	BREAKFAST	LUNCH	DINNER	SNACK
Monday	Baked Avocado Egg Boats	Pork and Mushroom Casserole	Chicken Moussaka	Mexican Cheese Poblanos
Tuesday	Baked Avocado Egg Boats	Lamb and Potato Casserole	Chicken and Artichoke Rice	Butter Cajun Shrimps
Wednesday	Baked Avocado Egg Boats	Pork and Mushroom Casserole	Easy Chicken Parmigiana	Three Cheese Nachos
Thursday	Baked Avocado Egg Boats	Cheese and Beef Meatballs	Basil and Minced Pork Fajita	Mexican Cheese Poblanos

Friday	Baked Avocado Egg Boats	Squash Quinoa Casserole	Shrimp Bibimbap	Tortilla Pocket
Saturday	Baked Avocado Egg Boats	Lamb and Potato Casserole	Classic Crab Cakes	Crispy Honey Chili Pork Tenderloins
Sunday	Baked Avocado Egg Boats	Pork and Mushroom Casserole	Chicken and Artichoke Rice	Chicken and Potato Taco

Chapter 2 Breakfast Recipes

1. Quick Sausage Cornmeal Pancakes

Preparation Time: 10 Minutes

Cooking Time: 20 Minutes

Servings: 5

Ingredients:

- 1 package gluten-free breakfast sausages.
- 1 cup cornmeal.
- 1 cup gluten-free all-purpose flour.
- 3 teaspoons gluten-free baking powder.
- ½ teaspoon baking soda.
- 1 teaspoon cinnamon.
- ¼ teaspoon nutmeg.
- ¼ teaspoon salt.
- 1 cup apple cider.
- ½ cup nonfat plain yogurt.
- 1 egg.
- 2 tablespoons maple syrup.
- 1 teaspoon vanilla.
- Butter, for greasing.
- ½ cup toasted pecans.
- Syrup, for serving

Directions:

1. Cook the sausages according to the package directions and then chop them into small pieces. Set aside.
2. In a large bowl, combine the cornmeal, flour, baking powder, baking soda, cinnamon, nutmeg and salt.
3. In another bowl, whisk together the apple cider, yogurt, egg, maple syrup, and vanilla.
4. Combine the wet and dry ingredients, including the sausages.
5. Heat a griddle or non-stick pan over medium heat. Coat the pan with butter and scoop about ⅓ cup of batter into the pan.
6. Cook each pancake for about 3 minutes, until the bottom is lightly browned, then flip to cook the other side for another 3 minutes.
7. Top with the toasted pecans and serve with syrup.

Nutrition:

Calories: 482 Cal

Fat: 24g

Carbs: 55g

Fiber: 6g

Protein: 17g

2. Berry Crepes

Preparation Time: 10 Minutes

Cooking Time: 20 Minutes

Servings: 4

Ingredients:

FOR THE CREPES

- 2 large eggs.
- ¾ cup milk.
- ½ cup water.
- 1 cup gluten-free all-purpose flour.
- ¼ teaspoon xanthan gum (leave out if your flour mix already has it).
- 3 tablespoons butter, melted.
- 2 tablespoons granulated sugar.
- 1 teaspoon pure vanilla extract.

FOR THE BERRY FILLING

- 2 cups mixed berries.
- ½ cup sugar.
- 1 tablespoon cornstarch.

FOR THE CREAM FILLING

- 1 cup heavy whipping cream.

- 1 cup sugar.

- 8 ounces cream cheese.

- 1 teaspoon vanilla extract.

TOPPING OPTIONS

- Mixed fresh berries.

- Powdered sugar.

Directions:

TO MAKE THE CREPES

1. Whisk the eggs in a large bowl, and then add the rest of the crepe ingredients and mix until smooth.

2. Heat a nonstick pan over medium-low heat. Pour ¼ cup of batter into the center of the pan. Pick up the pan and swirl it to spread the batter evenly, making a circle.

3. Cook over medium to medium-low heat for about 2 minutes, or until browned on the bottom.

4. Carefully flip the crepe over and cook the other side until golden brown. Repeat with the remaining batter. Stack the crepes on a plate and loosely cover with foil to keep them warm.

TO MAKE THE BERRY FILLING

- Once the crepes are done, mix the ingredients for the berry filling in a small saucepan and heat on medium-low until bubbly, about 10 minutes. Remove from heat and set aside.

TO MAKE THE CREAM FILLING

- Using a blender, whip the ingredients for the cream filling until thick and smooth, about 2 minutes.

TO ASSEMBLE THE CREPES

- Place a crepe on a plate. Top with berry and cream fillings. Roll the crepe up and top with more berry filling and fresh fruit.

Nutrition:

Calories: 989 Cal

Fat: 54g

Carbs: 120g

Fiber: 6g

Protein: 14g

3. Bacon and Cheese Frittata

Preparation Time: 5 Minutes

Cooking Time: 25 Minutes

Servings: 6

Ingredients:

- 1 teaspoon extra-virgin olive oil.
- 6 strips bacon.
- 6 large eggs.
- 1 cup whole milk.
- 2 tablespoons butter.
- Salt.
- Freshly ground black pepper.
- ¼ cup chopped scallions.
- 1 cup shredded Cheddar cheese.

Directions:

1. Preheat the oven to 350°F.
2. Grease an 11-by-7-inch baking dish with the oil.
3. Cook the bacon halfway (you don't want to cook it all the way because you still need to bake it) in the microwave, for about two minutes, and then chop it into bits and set aside.
4. In a large bowl, whisk together the eggs, milk, and butter, and season with salt and pepper. Pour the mixture into the

prepared baking dish. Sprinkle with the bacon, scallions, and cheese.

5. Bake for fifty-five minutes, or until the eggs are set.

Nutrition:

Calories: 256 Cal

Fat: 20g

Carbs: 3g

Fiber: 1g

Protein: 15g

4. Vegetable Frittata

Preparation Time: 10 Minutes

Cooking Time: 20 Minutes

Servings: 6

Ingredients:

- 2 tablespoons butter.
- 1 tablespoon extra-virgin olive oil.
- 1 red bell pepper, thinly sliced.
- 1 yellow bell pepper, thinly sliced.
- 1 red onion, cut into thin wedges.
- 1 small zucchini, cut lengthwise then cut diagonally.
- Salt.
- Freshly ground black pepper.
- 2 garlic cloves, minced.
- 3 or 4 scallions, chopped.
- 12 large eggs.
- 1 cup half and half.
- ¼ cup shredded Parmesan cheese.

Directions:

1. Preheat the oven to 350°F.
2. On the stovetop, heat a large cast-iron pan over medium-high heat. Heat the butter and oil, and then sauté the bell

peppers, red onion, and zucchini. Season with salt and pepper. Add the garlic and scallions, and sauté for another minute. Set aside.

3. Whisk the eggs, half-and-half, and Parmesan, and season with salt and pepper.

4. Pour the egg mixture into the pan with the sautéed vegetables. Stir to mix, and then bake for about 20 minutes, or until the eggs are set. Serve warm.

Nutrition:

Calories: 288 Cal

Fat: 21g

Carbs: 8g

Fiber: 2g

Protein: 16g

5. Egg Muffins

Preparation Time: 10 Minutes

Cooking Time: 20 Minutes

Servings: 12 Muffins

Ingredients:

- 1 tablespoon extra-virgin olive oil, plus more to grease the pan.
- ½ cup finely chopped onion.
- ¾ cup chopped cherry tomatoes.
- 12 eggs.
- 1 cup fresh baby spinach, roughly chopped.
- 1 cup milk.
- Pinch salt.
- Freshly ground black pepper.
- 1 ripe but firm avocado, peeled, pitted, and diced (optional).
- Fresh salsa (optional).
- 3 to 4 tablespoons crumbled feta cheese (optional).

Directions:

1. Preheat the oven to 350°F and grease a 12-muffin pan.
2. Heat the oil in a small pan over medium heat. Sauté the onions until soft and then add the tomatoes. Cook for a

couple of minutes, or until the tomatoes start to soften. Remove the pan from the heat and let it cool slightly.

3. In a large bowl, whisk together the eggs, spinach, and milk. Stir in the onion-and-tomato mixture, and then season with salt and pepper.

4. Carefully fill the muffin pan, allowing about half an inch for the eggs to expand while cooking.

5. Bake for about 20 minutes, or until eggs are set. Remove from the oven and let the muffins cool for a few minutes. If desired, serve with avocado, salsa, and feta cheese.

Nutrition:

Calories: 89 Cal

Fat: 6g

Carbs: 2g

Fiber: 1g

Protein: 7g

6. Baked Avocado Egg Boats

Preparation Time: 10 Minutes

Cooking Time: 12-15 Minutes

Servings: 4

Ingredients:

- 4 slices bacon.
- 2 ripe (semi-firm) avocados.
- 4 large eggs.
- 2 tablespoons finely chopped fresh chives.
- Salt.
- Freshly ground black pepper.

Directions:

1. Preheat the oven to 375°F.
2. Arrange the bacon strips on a paper towel–lined plate, and microwave until crispy, 3 to 5 minutes. Chop or crumble the bacon and set aside.
3. Slice the avocados in half and remove the pit. Scoop out about 2 tablespoons of avocado flesh to make the hole bigger to accommodate the egg. Place the avocados on an inverted muffin tin to keep them in place. Crack 1 egg into each avocado half and season with salt and pepper.
4. Bake for 12 to 15 minutes, or until eggs are set.
5. Garnish with the chives and crispy bacon.

Nutrition:

Calories: 260 Cal

Fat: 21g

Carbs: 8g

Fiber: 6g Protein: 12g

7. Berry-Chia Yogurt Parfait

Preparation Time: 10 Minutes

Cooking Time: 0 Minutes

Servings: 6 Cups

Ingredients:

- 2 cups mixed fresh berries, divided.
- 1 tablespoon agave nectar, divided.
- 3 cups plain yogurt.
- 1 cup gluten-free granola.
- 2 tablespoons chia seeds.

Directions:

1. In a large bowl, mix 1 cup of berries with ½ tablespoon of agave nectar and mash the berries to desired consistency. Add the remaining 1 cup of berries.
2. Combine the yogurt with the remaining ½ tablespoon of agave nectar in a medium bowl.

3. Spoon about 3 tablespoons of the yogurt mixture into six 8-ounce glasses. Top each glass with a few tablespoons of the berry mixture, and then sprinkle some of the granola and ½ teaspoon of chia seeds on top.
4. Repeat layers once.

Nutrition:

Calories: 191 Cal

Fat: 6g

Carbs: 26g

Fiber: 4g

Protein: 9g

8. Lean and Green Smoothie

Preparation Time: 10 Minutes

Cooking Time: 0 Minutes

Servings: 4 Cups

Ingredients:

- 1 Granny Smith apple.
- 2½ cups baby kale.
- 1 cup pineapple chunks.
- 1 cup apple juice, chilled.
- ½ cup green grapes, frozen.

135

Directions:

1. Peel, core, and chop the apple.
2. Place all the ingredients in a blender.
3. Cover and blend until smooth.

Nutrition:

Calories: 107 Cal

Fat: 1g

Carbs: 26g

Fiber: 4g

Protein: 2g

9. Hawaiian Smoothie Bowl

Preparation Time: 10 Minutes

Cooking Time: 0 Minutes

Servings: 4

Ingredients:

- 2 ripe bananas.

- 1½ cups frozen mango.

- 1½ cups frozen pineapple.

- 1 cup plain Greek yogurt.

- ¼ cup almond milk (add as needed).

Directions:

1. Combine the ingredients in a blender. Blend on high until smooth.

2. If the mixture is too thick, add a little bit of almond milk.

3. Pour into a serving bowl and top with your favorite fruits.

Nutrition:

Calories: 161 Cal

Fat: 2g

Carbs: 31g

Fiber: 3g

Protein: 7g

10. Chickpea Pancakes with maple Yogurt Topping and Berries

Preparation Time: 15 Minutes

Cooking Time: 20 Minutes

Servings: 4

Ingredients:

FOR THE PANCAKES

- 1 cup chickpea flour.
- ½ cup potato starch.
- 2½ teaspoons baking powder.
- ¼ teaspoon salt (preferably pink Himalayan).
- 2 large eggs.
- 1 cup nondairy milk.
- 2 tablespoons extra-virgin olive oil.
- 1 tablespoon maple syrup.
- 1 tablespoon distilled white vinegar.

FOR THE TOPPING

- 1 cup non-dairy vanilla yogurt.
- 2 tablespoons maple syrup.
- ¼ teaspoon ground cinnamon.
- 1 cup fresh berries, such as blueberries, raspberries, or chopped strawberries.

138

Directions:

TO MAKE THE PANCAKES

1. In a large bowl, combine the flour, potato starch, baking powder, and salt.
2. In a small bowl, whisk together the eggs, milk, oil, maple syrup, and vinegar. Pour over the flour mixture and stir just until combined. Let stand for 5 minutes. The batter may be slightly lumpy.
3. Lightly coat a griddle with nonstick cooking spray. Heat over medium heat.
4. Reduce the heat under the griddle to medium-low. Drop a scant ¼ cup of batter onto the griddle. Cook for 2 to 3 minutes, or until bubbles form. Flip and cook 2 minutes longer, or until golden brown. Repeat this process with the remaining batter.

TO MAKE THE TOPPING

1. In a small bowl, whisk together the yogurt, maple syrup and cinnamon.
2. Serve the pancakes warm with yogurt topping and fresh berries.

Nutrition:

Calories: 335 Cal

Fat: 14g

Carbs: 45g

Fiber: 4g

Protein: 9g

Chapter 3 Other Breakfast Recipes

11. Tropical Pineapple Green Smoothie

Preparation Time: 5 Minutes Cooking Time: 0 Minute

Servings: 1

Ingredients:

- 2 cups packed baby spinach.
- 1 cup frozen pineapple cubes.
- ½ banana, sliced and frozen.
- ½ avocado.
- ½ to ¾ cup coconut water.

Directions:

1. In a blender, combine the spinach, pineapple, banana, avocado, and ½ cup coconut water. Process until smooth and add up to ¼ cup more coconut water if needed.

Nutrition:

Calories: 316 Cal

Fat: 14g

Carbs: 49g

Fiber: 12g

Protein: 6g

12. Fluffy Scrambled Eggs, Sausage, Spinach, and Mushroom Bowl

Preparation Time: 10 Minutes

Cooking Time: 15 Minutes

Servings: 4

Ingredients:

- 4 ounces bulk turkey sausage.
- ½ teaspoon ground cumin.
- 2 cups packed baby spinach.
- 2 cups diced mushrooms.
- 1 scallion, white and green parts, thinly sliced.
- 2 tablespoons extra-virgin olive oil, divided.
- ½ teaspoon salt (preferably pink Himalayan), divided.
- 6 large eggs.
- 2 tablespoons non-dairy milk.
- Freshly ground black pepper.
- 1 tablespoon chopped fresh basil.
- Salsa or ketchup, for topping (optional).
- Fresh avocado slices, for topping (optional).

Directions:

1. In a large nonstick skillet, cook the sausage and cumin over medium-high heat for 5 to 7 minutes, or until cooked through, breaking into tiny pieces with a wooden spoon. When fully cooked, add the spinach, mushrooms, and scallion and cook for 4 to 5 minutes, or until tender, adding 1 tablespoon of oil if necessary.
2. Stir in ¼ teaspoon of salt. Cover and set aside.
3. In a large bowl, whisk together the eggs, milk, remaining ¼ teaspoon of salt, and pepper to taste for 30 seconds. This gets air flowing through and makes the eggs fluffy.
4. In a medium skillet, heat the remaining 1 tablespoon of olive oil over medium-low heat. Add the eggs and let sit for 1 minute without stirring. Then, with a wooden spoon or heatproof spatula, stir the eggs constantly until fully cooked.
5. Remove from the heat and fold in the basil and the sausage mixture.
6. Serve topped with salsa or ketchup and fresh avocado slices (if using).

Nutrition:

Calories: 199 Cal

Fat: 16g

Carbs: 3g

Fiber: 1g

Protein: 13g

13. Chocolate Chip Banana Bread Loaf

Preparation Time: 15 Minutes

Cooking Time: 55 Minutes

Servings: 1 Loaf

Ingredients:

- 3 ripe bananas.
- 2 cups all-purpose gluten-free flour.
- 1 tablespoon baking powder.
- 1 teaspoon ground cinnamon.
- ½ teaspoon salt (preferably pink Himalayan).
- 2 large eggs.
- ⅔ Cup maple syrup.
- ½ cup nondairy yogurt.
- 1 tablespoon vanilla extract.
- 1 cup dairy-free mini chocolate chips.

Directions:

1. Preheat the oven to 350°F. Line a 9-inch loaf pan with parchment paper so there is an overhang on two long sides.

2. In a small bowl, mash the bananas with a fork until creamy and blended.

3. In a medium bowl, combine the flour, baking powder, cinnamon, and salt.

4. In a large bowl, using an electric mixer beat the eggs, maple syrup, yogurt, and vanilla on medium speed until well blended. Beat in the mashed bananas until combined. On low speed, beat in the flour mixture just until combined. Fold in ¾ cup of chocolate chips. Spoon the batter into the prepared pan. Sprinkle the remaining ¼ cup of chocolate chips over the top.

5. Bake for 50 to 60 minutes, or until a toothpick inserted in the center comes out clean. Let cool in the pan on a wire rack for 20 minutes, then remove by lifting the parchment paper. Transfer to the rack to cool completely. Wrap and store overnight for best slicing.

Nutrition:

Calories: 265 Cal

Fat: 7g

Carbs: 52g

Fiber: 3g

Protein: 5g

14. Chocolate Chip Oatmeal Chia Seed Muffins

Preparation Time: 10 Minutes

Cooking Time: 20 Minutes

Servings: 12 Muffins

Ingredients:

- 2 large eggs.
- ½ cup honey.
- ¼ cup coconut oil, melted.
- 1 teaspoon vanilla extract.
- 1 cup all-purpose gluten-free flour.
- 1 cup gluten-free quick-cooking oats.
- ¼ cup flaxseed meal.
- 2 tablespoons chia seeds.
- 1 teaspoon ground cinnamon.
- 1 teaspoon baking powder.
- ½ teaspoon baking soda.
- ½ teaspoon salt (preferably pink Himalayan).
- ½ cup unsweetened almond milk or coconut milk beverage.
- 1 cup dairy-free chocolate chips.

Directions:

1. Preheat the oven to 350°F. Line a muffin pan with paper liners and coat the liners with nonstick cooking spray.
2. In a small bowl, whisk together the eggs, honey, coconut oil, and vanilla.
3. In a medium bowl, stir together the flour, oats, flaxseed meal, chia seeds, cinnamon, baking powder, baking soda, and salt. Pour the egg mixture into the flour mixture. Add the almond milk and stir together until well combined.
4. Carefully fold in the chocolate chips.
5. Evenly divide the mixture into the prepared muffin cups. Bake for 20 to 22 minutes, or until the tops are slightly browned. Let cool in the pan on a wire rack for 10 minutes, then transfer to the rack to cool completely. These muffins are best consumed within 3 days after baking.

Nutrition:

Calories: 292 Cal

Fat: 14g

Carbs: 41g

Fiber: 3g

Protein: 6g

15. Blueberry Oatmeal Muffins

Preparation Time: 10 Minutes

Cooking Time: 20 Minutes

Servings: 12 Muffins

Ingredients:

- 1 cup all-purpose gluten-free flour.
- 1 cup gluten-free rolled oats.
- 1 teaspoon baking powder.
- ½ teaspoon baking soda.
- ¾ teaspoon salt (preferably pink Himalayan).
- 2 large eggs.
- ⅔ Cup maple syrup.
- ½ cup nondairy yogurt.
- ¼ cup coconut oil, melted.
- ¼ cup nondairy milk.
- 1 teaspoon grated lemon zest.
- 1 teaspoon vanilla extract.
- 1 cup blueberries.

Directions:

1. Preheat the oven to 350°F. Line a muffin pan with paper liners and coat the liners with nonstick cooking spray.

2. In a large bowl, whisk together the flour, oats, baking powder, baking soda, and salt.

3. In a medium bowl, whisk together the eggs, maple syrup, yogurt, oil, milk, lemon zest, and vanilla until blended. Fold the egg mixture into the flour mixture just until moistened. Carefully fold in the blueberries. Let the batter stand for 5 minutes to soak the oats.

4. Evenly divide the mixture into the prepared muffin cups. Bake for 20 minutes, or until golden on top and a toothpick inserted in the center of a muffin comes out clean. Remove the muffins from the pan and transfer to a cooling rack to cool completely.

Nutrition:

Calories: 185 Cal

Fat: 7g

Carbs: 28g

Fiber: 1g

Protein: 4g

16. Peanut Butter and Chocolate Swirl Overnight Oats

Preparation Time: 10 Minutes + Overnight Set

Cooking Time: 0 Minutes

Servings: 4

Ingredients:

- 2 cups gluten-free rolled oats.
- 2 cups nondairy milk, plus more for serving.
- Salt (preferably Pink Himalayan).
- 4 tablespoons organic peanut butter.
- 4 tablespoons unsweetened cocoa powder.
- 4 tablespoons honey or maple syrup.
- 2 teaspoons ground cinnamon.
- 4 tablespoons chopped peanuts or pecans.

Directions:

1. In each of four 16-ounce mason jars with lids, combine ½ cup of oats and ½ cup of milk. Mix until the oats are well coated. Sprinkle each with a dash of salt.
2. Top each jar with 1 tablespoon of peanut butter, 1 tablespoon of cocoa powder, 1 tablespoon of honey, and ½ teaspoon of cinnamon. Mix well.
3. Cover each jar with a lid and let it stand in the refrigerator overnight.

4. To serve, top each jar with 1 tablespoon of chopped nuts and extra milk. Enjoy chilled or warm.

Nutrition:

Calories: 446 Cal

Fat: 18g

Carbs: 61g

Fiber: 9g Protein: 18g

17. Sun-Dried Tomato Basil Frittata Muffins

Preparation Time: 15 Minutes

Cooking Time: 15 Minutes

Servings: 12 Muffins

Ingredients:

- 12 large eggs.
- ¼ teaspoon salt (preferably pink Himalayan).
- ¼ teaspoon freshly ground black pepper.
- 1 cup packed baby spinach, finely chopped.
- ½ cup sun-dried tomatoes in olive oil, drained and chopped.
- 5 tablespoons green olive slices.
- 1 scallion, green parts only, sliced.
- 1 garlic clove, minced.

- 2 tablespoons chopped fresh basil, divided.

Directions:

1. Preheat the oven to 350°F. Coat a silicone muffin pan with nonstick cooking spray or line a regular muffin pan with paper liners and coat the liners with nonstick cooking spray. Please note that this recipe works best with a silicone muffin pan.
2. In a large bowl, whisk together the eggs, salt, and pepper, getting air throughout the eggs. This makes the eggs fluffy.
3. Stir in the spinach, sun-dried tomatoes, olives, scallion, garlic, and 1 tablespoon of basil.
4. Evenly divide the mixture into the prepared muffin cups. Bake for 15 to 20 minutes, or until the centers are set. Let stand for about 5 minutes before serving. Remove from the pan and garnish with the remaining 1 tablespoon of basil. If desired, sprinkle with salt and pepper to taste.

Nutrition: Calories: 91 Cal

Fat: 5g

Carbs: 4g

Fiber: 2g

Protein: 6g

18. Acai Smoothie Bowl

Preparation Time: 15 Minutes

Cooking Time: 0 Minutes

Servings: 2

Ingredients:

- 2 (3.5-ounce) packs frozen acai smoothie puree.
- 1 cup frozen sliced strawberries.
- 1 banana, fresh or frozen.
- ¼ cup fresh spinach.
- ½ to ¾ cup apple juice.

TOPPINGS (OPTIONAL)

- Banana slices.
- Sliced strawberries.
- Raspberries.
- Blueberries.
- Chopped nuts and seeds.
- Hemp seeds.
- Chia seeds.
- Honey.

Directions:

1. In a blender or food processor, combine the acai smoothie puree, strawberries, banana, spinach, and ½ cup of apple juice. Blend until smooth, adding more apple juice if needed. It should be very thick in consistency, but smooth, with no visible chunks. Divide between two bowls and sprinkle with the toppings of your choice (if using).

Nutrition:

Calories: 175 Cal

Fat: 6g

Carbs: 30g

Fiber: 5g

Protein: 2g

19. Honey-Nut Granola

Preparation Time: 10 Minutes

Cooking Time: 20 Minutes

Servings: 5

Ingredients:

- 3 cups gluten-free rolled oats.
- ¾ cup unsalted cashew pieces.
- ¾ cup slivered almonds.
- ½ cup honey.
- 7 tablespoons coconut oil, melted (or non-dairy butter, melted).
- 1 teaspoon vanilla extract.
- ¼ teaspoon salt (preferably pink Himalayan).
- ⅓ Cup dried fruit, such as raisins or cranberries.

Directions:

1. Preheat the oven to 325°F. Line a baking sheet with parchment paper.
2. In a large bowl, combine the oats, cashews, and almonds. Add the honey, oil, vanilla, and salt and toss to coat well.
3. Spread onto the prepared baking sheet. Bake for 25 to 30 minutes, or until golden brown, stirring occasionally to prevent burning. Set the pan on a wire rack to cool and immediately stir in the dried fruit.

4. Let cool to harden, then break into chunks before serving or storing. Store in an airtight container in a cool dry place.

Nutrition:

Calories: 353 Cal

Fat: 20g

Carbs: 40g

Fiber: 4g

Protein: 7g

Chapter 4 Lunch Recipes

20. Mediterranean Lamb Casserole

Preparation Time: 15 Minutes

Cooking Time: 10 Minutes

Servings: 5

Ingredients:

- 2 lb. boned lean shoulder of lamb.
- 3 onions, sliced.
- 2 garlic cloves, chopped.
- 1 15 oz. can chickpeas, drained and rinsed.
- 2 zucchinis, peeled and cubed.
- 1 cup cherry tomatoes, halved.
- 1 cup beef broth.
- 1 cup tomato juice.
- 3 tbsp. olive oil.
- 1 tbsp. fresh rosemary, chopped.
- 1 tbsp. fresh basil, chopped.
- ½ tsp. black pepper.
- ½ cup fresh parsley leaves, to serve.

Directions:

1. Cut the lamb into 1-inch cubes.

2. In an ovenproof casserole, heat 2 tablespoons of the olive oil and gently sauté onions and garlic for about 2-3 minutes.
3. Add the lamb and sauté, stirring, for about 4 minutes or until well browned on all sides.
4. Add in rosemary, tomato juice and beef broth and bake in a preheated to 350°F for 1 hour.
5. Stir in the chickpeas and bake for a further 1 hour or until the lamb is almost tender.
6. Stir in zucchinis, tomatoes, black pepper and basil. Cook for about 20 minutes longer or until the lamb is tender.
7. Serve sprinkled with parsley.

Nutrition:

Calories: 344 Cal

Fat: 5g

Carbs: 17g

Fiber: 3g

Protein: 7g

21. Lamb and Potato Casserole

Preparation Time: 15 Minutes

Cooking Time: 10 Minutes

Servings: 6

Ingredients:

- 2 pounds shoulder lamb chops.
- 15 small new potatoes, peeled, whole.
- 3 large onions, sliced.
- 2 carrots, sliced.
- 2 tbsp. olive oil.
- 2 tsp. dried parsley.
- 2 tsp. dried mint.
- ½ tsp. black pepper.
- ½ tsp. salt.

Directions:

1. Place the lamb chops into a greased casserole dish. Cover them with sliced onion, carrots, parsley, salt and pepper.
2. Arrange new potatoes on and around the meat.
3. Add enough cold water to fill the dish halfway.
4. Bake, covered with foil, for 45 minutes in a preheated oven.
5. Remove the foil and bake for 30 minutes more.

Nutrition:

Calories: 269 Cal

Fat: 11g

Carbs: 18g

Fiber: 3g

Protein: 25g

22. Pork and Mushroom Casserole

Preparation Time: 15 Minutes

Cooking Time: 10 Minutes

Servings: 4

Ingredients:

- 2 lb. pork loin, cut into cubes.
- 1 large onion, chopped.
- 1 carrot, chopped.
- 2 cups mushrooms, cut.
- 3 tbsp. olive oil.
- 1/3 cup sour cream.
- Salt and black pepper, to taste.

Directions:

1. Heat the olive oil in a casserole dish and seal the pork cubes for about 5 minutes, stirring continuously. Lower the heat, add the onion and carrot and sauté for 3-4 minutes until the onion is soft.
2. Cover with a lid or foil and simmer for 1 hour at 350°F, or until the pork is tender. Uncover, add the sour cream, salt and pepper to taste, stir, and bake for 10 minutes more. Serve with boiled potatoes or gluten-free pasta.

Nutrition:

Calories: 263 Cal

Fat: 11g

Carbs: 15g

Fiber: 2g

Protein: 25g

23. Pork Roast and Cabbage

Preparation Time: 15 Minutes

Cooking Time: 10 Minutes

Servings: 4

Ingredients:

- 2 cups of cooked pork roast, chopped.
- 1/2 head of cabbage, chopped.
- 2 onions, chopped.
- 1 lemon, juice only.
- 1 tomato, chopped.
- 1 tsp. paprika.
- 1/2 tsp. cumin.
- Black pepper, to taste.
- 2 tbsp. olive oil.

Directions:

1. Heat olive oil in an ovenproof casserole and sauté cabbage, pork and onions.
2. Add cumin, paprika, lemon juice, tomato and stir. Cover and bake at 350 F until vegetables are tender.

Nutrition:

Calories: 291 Cal

Fat: 18g

Carbs: 28g

Fiber: 1g

Protein: 23g

24. Korean-Style Honeyed Chicken

Preparation Time: 1 Minute

Cooking Time: 10 Minutes

Servings: 4

Ingredients:

- 1 whole chicken, about 5-6 pounds 2 teaspoons sea salt.
- 4 teaspoons turmeric, ground.
- 4 teaspoons chili powder.
- 4 teaspoons black pepper, ground ¼ cup onion, diced.
- ½ cup garlic, minced.
- 3 tablespoons honey. ¼ cup brown sugar.

164

- 2 tablespoons olive or vegetable oil.

Directions:

1. Mix the salt, turmeric, chili powder, black pepper, and brown sugar in a small bowl.
2. Rub the chicken skin with the mixture.
3. Spread the oil over the bottom of the slow cooker. Place the chicken breast-side up in the slow cooker and surround it with onion, garlic, and honey.
4. Cook for 10 Minutes on low.
5. Check to ensure that the chicken is cooked. The juice should run clear when poked with a fork in the thigh. The temperature on a meat thermometer should read 165°F when inserted in the thickest part of the breast without touching any bones.

Nutrition:

Calories: 215 Cal

Fat: 3g

Carbs: 9g

Fiber: 1g Protein: 36g

25. Cheese and Beef Meatballs

Preparation Time: 15 Minutes

Cooking Time: 7 Minutes

Servings: 4-6

Ingredients:

- 20 gluten-free frozen beef meatballs 2 tablespoons olive oil.
- 1 6 oz. can of tomato paste.
- 1 cup tomato sauce.
- 2 teaspoons chili powder.
- 2 teaspoons paprika.
- 1 cup beef broth.
- ¾ cup grated cheddar cheese.

Directions:

1. Sprinkle black pepper over the meatballs.
2. Place the meatballs, olive oil, tomato paste, tomato sauce, chili powder, paprika powder, and broth in slow cooker.
3. Cook for 6 Minutes on low.
4. Sprinkle cheddar cheese on top and cook for 1 more minute.

Nutrition:

Calories: 131 Cal

Fat: 5g

Carbs: 18g

Fiber: 6g

Protein: 5g

26. Creamy Corn and Pork Bits

Preparation Time: 15 Minutes

Cooking Time: 7 Minutes

Servings: 8

Ingredients:

- 2 pounds ground pork.
- 1 ½ cups corn kernels, frozen or canned 1 cup milk.
- ½ cup sour cream, plus extra for serving 5 teaspoons butter, melted.
- 1 tablespoon honey.
- 2 tablespoons fresh chives, chopped (or 1 tablespoon dried chives) Salt and pepper.

Directions:

1. Place ground pork in a skillet and brown. Drain the fat.
2. Add the pork to the slow cooker, and add the corn, milk, sour cream, butter, honey, and chives.
3. Set the slow cooker to low and cook for 7 Minutes.
4. Top with a dollop of sour cream before serving.

Nutrition:

Calories: 160 Cal

Fat: 6g

Carbs: 22g

Fiber: 2g

Protein: 8g

27. Squash Quinoa Casserole

Preparation Time: 15 Minutes

Cooking Time: 7 Minutes

Servings: 4

Ingredients:

- 12 ounces of tomatillos, de-husked and chopped.
- 1 pint of cherry tomatoes, chopped.
- 1 bell pepper, chopped.
- ½ cup of chopped onion.
- 1 tablespoon of lime juice.
- 1 teaspoon of salt.
- 1 cup of quinoa.
- 1 cup of feta cheese.
- 2 pounds of yellow squash, sliced.
- 2 tablespoons of oregano.

Directions:

1. Chop everything up that needs to get cut.

2. Place everything in the crock pot and cook on low for four Minutes.

3. Serve and enjoy.

Nutrition:

Calories: 184 Cal

Fat: 4g

Carbs: 34g

Fiber: 5g

Protein: 6g

28. Pinto Bean Sloppy Joe Mix

Preparation Time: 15 Minutes

Cooking Time: 7 Minutes

Servings: 4

Ingredients:

- 2 tablespoons of olive oil.
- 2 carrots, sliced.
- 1 onion, sliced.
- 4 cloves of garlic, minced.
- 3 tablespoons of chili powder.
- 2 tablespoons of balsamic vinegar.
- 1 cup of pinto beans.

- 1 red bell pepper, diced.
- 8 ounces of tomato sauce.
- ½ cup of water.
- 2 tablespoons of gluten-free soy sauce.
- 2 tablespoons of tomato paste.
- 4 cups of green cabbage, sliced.
- 1 zucchini, chopped.
- 1 cup of corn.
- 3 tablespoons of honey mustard.
- 1 tablespoon of brown sugar.
- 1 teaspoon of salt.
- 10 lettuce leaves.

Directions:

1. Cut up everything that needs to get cut up and place in slow cooker.
2. Cook on high heat for 5 Minutes with the other ingredients.
3. Place the cabbage and the zucchini in the last 30 minutes.
4. Serve on lettuce and enjoy.

Nutrition:

Calories: 144 Cal

Fat: 1g

Carbs: 26g

Fiber: 3g

Protein: 8g

29. Turkey Stew with Green Chilies

Preparation Time: 15 Minutes

Cooking Time: 7 Minutes

Servings: 4

Ingredients:

- 1 ½ cups butternut squash (peeled and diced).
- 1 lb. /500 g ground turkey.
- 2 large potatoes (peeled and diced).
- 3 medium carrots (peeled and chopped).
- 1 onion (diced).
- 4 cloves garlic (minced).
- 1 teaspoon cumin.
- 1 teaspoon chili powder.
- 1 cup roasted chopped green chili.
- 1-quart gluten-free chicken stock.
- Low salt and black pepper to taste.

Directions:

1. First, brown the ground turkey in a skillet and take out the excess fat, if any.

2. Now add the turkey to the slow cooker with the remaining ingredients up to salt and black pepper. Stir well to combine.
3. Cover and cook until the pork is done.
4. About 20 minutes before serving, stir in the lime juice and cilantro. Add some sweetener, if needed, to balance out the spice and if you need a little more liquid, add more broth to it and heat through.

Nutrition:

Calories: 122 Cal

Fat: 1g

Carbs: 15g

Fiber: 3g

Protein: 12g

30. Mushroom Tomato with Onion Gravy

Preparation Time: 5 Minutes

Cooking Time: 25 Minutes

Servings: 4

Ingredients:

- 1 pound mushroom.
- 8 onions, chopped.
- 2 tbsp. of olive oil.
- 3 red chilies, chopped.
- ½ cup of water.
- 2 green chilies, chopped.
- 4 tomatoes, chopped.
- 1 tsp. of ginger.
- Fresh parsley.
- 1 tsp. garlic.
- Salt and pepper to taste.

Directions:

1. In a pan heat the oil.
2. Stir in the onions and toss for about 3 minutes or until they are brown.
3. Stir in the mushrooms and toss for 6-8 minutes.
4. Now stir in the green chilies, and all spices.

5. Season with salt and toss for about 10 minutes.

6. Sprinkle the parsley and then serve.

Nutrition:

Calories: 163 Cal

Fat: 3g

Carbs: 8g

Fiber: 2g

Protein: 24g

31. Greek Chicken Salad

Preparation Time: 15 Minutes

Cooking Time: 7 Minutes

Servings: 4

Ingredients:

- 4 small chicken breast halves
- 1/3 cup lemon juice.
- 1-2 tsp. chopped fresh rosemary.
- 3 garlic cloves, crushed.
- 1/4 cup olive oil.
- 2 tomatoes cut into thin wedges.
- 1 small red onion, cut into thin wedges.
- 1/4 cup black olives.
- 3.5 oz. feta, crumbled.
- 1/4 cup parsley leaves, chopped.

Directions:

1. Prepare the dressing from the lemon juice, garlic, rosemary and olive oil.
2. Place the chicken breasts in a bowl with half the dressing. Stir well and marinate for at least fifteen minutes.
3. Heat a chargrill pan or non-stick frying pan over medium-high heat.

4. Cook the chicken for five minutes each side until golden and cooked through.

5. Set aside, covered with foil.

6. Toss the tomatoes, onion, olives, feta and parsley in the remaining dressing.

7. Slice the chicken thickly and add to the salad, then toss gently to combine.

Nutrition:

Calories: 255 Cal

Fat: 13g

Carbs: 11g

Fiber: 3g

Protein: 24g

Chapter 5 Lunch Recipes

32. Turkey Quinoa Salad

Preparation Time: 15 Minutes

Cooking Time: 10 Minutes

Servings: 4

Ingredients:

- 1 cup quinoa.
- 2 cups water.
- 1 cup skinless lean turkey breast, cooked, diced.
- 1 small red onion, chopped.
- 2 carrots diced and cooked.
- 1 cup green peas, cooked.
- 2 tbsp. olive oil.
- 1 tbsp. lemon juice.
- Salt and black pepper, to taste.

Directions:

1. Wash quinoa with lots of water. Strain it and cook it according to package directions.
2. When ready, set aside in a large salad bowl and fluff with a fork.
3. Add turkey, onion, carrots and green peas.

4. Combine oil, lemon juice, salt and pepper in a separate bowl and stir until well mixed.

5. Pour dressing over quinoa mixture and stir again.

6. Cover and chill until ready to serve.

Nutrition:

Calories: 255 Cal

Fat: 2g

Carbs: 35g

Fiber: 6g

Protein: 26g

33. Tuna and Green Bean Salad

Preparation Time: 15 Minutes

Cooking Time: 10 Minutes

Servings: 4

Ingredients:

- 3 boiled potatoes cut.
- 9 oz. green beans, trimmed and cut into 2-inch lengths.
- 2 tomatoes, sliced.
- A bunch of baby rocket leaves.
- 1 Can tuna, drained and broken into big chunks.
- 1/4 cup olive oil.
- 2 tbsp. lemon juice.
- 3 tbsp. homemade pesto.

Directions:

1. Boil the green beans for 5-6 minutes. Drain and set aside to cool.
2. Prepare the dressing by combining olive oil, lemon juice and pesto. Season with salt and black pepper to taste.
3. Combine potatoes, green beans, tomatoes, baby rocket, tuna and the dressing.
4. Toss gently and serve.

Nutrition:

Calories: 237 Cal

Fat: 13g

Carbs: 19g

Fiber: 10g

Protein: 15g

34. Greek Chicken Casserole

Preparation Time: 15 Minutes

Cooking Time: 45 Minutes

Servings: 5-6

Ingredients:

- 4 skinless, boneless chicken breast halves or 8 tights.
- 2 lb. potatoes, cubed.
- 1 lb. green beans, trimmed and cut in 1-inch pieces.
- 1 big onion, chopped.
- 1 cup diced tomatoes.
- 5 cloves garlic, minced.
- 1/4 cup water.
- ½ cup feta cheese, crumbled.
- Salt and black pepper, to taste.

Directions:

1. Preheat oven to 350°F. Heat oil in a large baking dish over medium heat.
2. Add onion and sauté for 2 minutes. Add thyme, black pepper and garlic and sauté for another minute.
3. Add potatoes and sauté, for 2-3 minutes, or until they begin to brown. Stir in beans, water and tomatoes.
4. Remove from heat. Arrange chicken pieces into the vegetables, sprinkle with salt and pepper and top with feta.
5. Cover and bake for 40 minutes, stirring gently halfway through.
6. Serve the vegetable mixture on a plate underneath or beside the chicken.

Nutrition:

Calories: 123 Cal

Fat: 3g

Carbs: 18g

Fiber: 5g

Protein: 8g

35. Hunter Style Chicken

Preparation Time: 10 Minutes

Cooking Time: 40 Minutes

Servings: 4-6

Ingredients:

- 1 chicken (about 3 lbs.), cut into pieces.
- 2 onions, thinly sliced.
- 1-2 red bell peppers, chopped.
- 6-7 white mushrooms, sliced.
- 2 cups canned tomatoes, diced and drained.
- 3 garlic cloves, thinly sliced.
- Salt and freshly ground pepper, to taste.
- 1/3 cup white wine.
- ½ cup parsley leaves, finely cut.
- 1 bay leaf.
- 1 tsp. sugar.
- 2 tbsp. olive oil.

Directions:

1. Rinse chicken pieces and pat dry. Heat olive oil in a large skillet on medium heat. Working in batches, cook the chicken pieces until nicely browned. Transfer chicken to a bowl and set aside. Add 2 tbsp. of olive oil and sauté the

sliced onions and bell peppers for a few minutes. Add the mushrooms and cook some more until onion is translucent. Add in garlic and cook a minute more.

2. Add wine and simmer until liquid is reduced by half. Add tomatoes and a teaspoon of sugar and stir. Place chicken and the tomato mixture in an ovenproof casserole dish and bake in a preheated to 350°F oven for 35-40 minutes.

Nutrition:

Calories: 185 Cal

Fat: 12g

Carbs: 5g

Fiber: 1g

Protein: 13g

36. Chicken with Almonds and Prunes

Preparation Time: 8 Minutes

Cooking Time: 10 Minutes

Servings: 4

Ingredients:

- 1.5 lb. chicken thigh fillets, trimmed.
- ½ cup fresh orange juice.
- 2 tbsp. honey.
- 1/3 cup white wine.
- ½ cup pitted prunes.
- 2 tbsp. blanched almonds.
- 2 tbsp. raisins or sultanas.
- 1 tsp. ground cinnamon.
- Salt and ground black pepper, to taste.
- 1 tbsp. fresh parsley leaves, chopped.

Directions:

1. Combine orange juice, wine, honey, prunes, almonds, raisins and cinnamon in a large saucepan. Bring to a boil, reduce heat to medium and boil for 5-8 minutes or until liquid is reduced by 1/3.
2. Add the chicken thigh fillets and simmer over low heat, for 10 minutes, or until chicken is just tender. Season to taste with salt and pepper. Serve sprinkled with parsley.

Nutrition:

Calories: 234 Cal

Fat: 11g

Carbs: 12g

Fiber: 3g

Protein: 23g

37. Lemon Rosemary Chicken

Preparation Time: 15 Minutes

Cooking Time: 45 Minutes

Servings: 4

Ingredients:

- 4 boneless skinless chicken breasts or 4-5 tights.
- 2 garlic cloves, crushed.
- 4-5 lemon slices.
- 4-5 black olives, pitted.
- 1 tbsp. capers.
- 1 tbsp. dried rosemary.
- 3 tbsp. olive oil.
- Salt and pepper, to taste.

Directions:

1. Place the lemon slices at the bottom of a skillet and lay the chicken breasts on top of the lemon. Add in olives, rosemary, capers, salt and pepper to taste.
2. Cover, and cook, on medium-low, for 35-40 minutes or until the chicken is cooked through.
3. Uncover and cook for 2-3 minutes, until the liquid evaporates.

Nutrition:

Calories: 191 Cal

Fat: 2g

Carbs: 11g

Fiber: 1g

Protein: 31g

Chapter 6 Dinner Recipes

38. Baja Fish Tacos

Preparation Time: 15 Minutes

Cooking Time: 8 Minutes

Servings: 4

Ingredients:

- 2 tablespoons extra-virgin olive oil.
- Zest of 1 lime.
- Juice of 1 lime.
- 1 teaspoon ground cumin.
- 1 teaspoon ancho chile powder.
- ¼ teaspoon sea salt.
- ⅛ Teaspoon cayenne pepper.
- 1 pound mahi mahi, cut into 4-inch-long pieces.
- ½ cup mayonnaise.
- ½ cup sour cream
- ¼ cup minced fresh cilantro.
- 16 gluten-free corn tortillas.
- 1 cup shredded cabbage.
- ½ red onion, thinly sliced.
- 1 cup store-bought gluten-free roasted tomato salsa.

Directions:

1. In a large, nonreactive dish, whisk the olive oil, lime zest, lime juice, cumin, ancho chile powder, salt, and cayenne pepper. Add the mahi mahi to this mixture, turn to coat, and refrigerate for 10 minutes.
2. In a small jar, whisk the mayonnaise, sour cream, and cilantro. Cover and refrigerate until ready to serve.
3. Heat a large skillet or sauté pan over medium-high heat until hot. Remove the mahi mahi from the marinade, add to the skillet, and panfry for 3 to 4 minutes on each side, or until it flakes easily with a fork.
4. Evenly divide the fish among the tortillas. Top each taco with some shredded cabbage, onion, and salsa. Finish with a dollop of the cilantro sauce.

Nutrition:

Calories: 602 Cal

Fat: 27g

Carbs: 58g

Fiber: 8g

Protein: 36g

39. Classic Crab Cakes

Preparation Time: 5 Minutes

Cooking Time: 10 Minutes

Servings: 2-4

Ingredients:

- 1 scallion, white and green parts, thinly sliced.
- 1 teaspoon minced garlic.
- ½ cup gluten-free bread crumbs.
- 1 egg.
- 2 tablespoons mayonnaise.
- 1 teaspoon Old Bay Seasoning.
- 1 pound lump crabmeat, picked over for shells.
- Sea salt.
- Freshly ground black pepper.
- 2 tablespoons extra-virgin olive oil.

Directions:

1. In a medium bowl, combine the scallion, garlic, bread crumbs, egg, mayonnaise, and Old Bay Seasoning. Whisk until thoroughly combined.
2. Fold in the crabmeat, trying not to break up the larger pieces of crab. Season with salt and pepper. Form the crab mixture into 6 individual cakes.

3. Heat a large skillet or sauté pan over medium-high heat until hot. Add the olive oil and tilt the pan to coat the bottom.
4. Cook the crab cakes for 4 to 5 minutes on each side, until they're golden brown.

Nutrition:

Calories: 551 Cal

Fat: 27g

Carbs: 24g

Fiber: 2g

Protein: 53g

40. Shrimp Bibimbap

Preparation Time: 10 Minutes

Cooking Time: 20 Minutes

Servings: 4

Ingredients:

- 1½ cups white rice.
- 2 cups water.
- Sea salt.
- 1 teaspoon minced peeled fresh ginger.
- 1 teaspoon minced garlic.
- 2 tablespoons gluten-free soy sauce, plus more for serving.
- 1 tablespoon Sriracha chili sauce.
- 1 tablespoon plus 1 teaspoon toasted sesame oil, divided.
- 1 tablespoon freshly squeezed lime juice.
- 1 tablespoon honey.
- 1 pound large shrimp, peeled and deveined.
- 4 cups fresh spinach.
- 1 cup sliced button mushrooms.
- 1 tablespoon canola oil.
- 4 eggs.
- 2 tablespoons toasted sesame seeds.
- 1 cup kimchee (optional).

Directions:

1. In a medium pot over medium-high heat, bring the rice, water, and a generous pinch salt to a simmer. Cover and cook on low for about 20 minutes, until the rice is tender.

2. While the rice cooks, in a small nonreactive bowl, whisk the ginger, garlic, soy sauce, Sriracha, 1 tablespoon of the sesame oil, lime juice, and honey. Let the sauce rest for 5 minutes.

3. In a large skillet or sauté pan over medium heat, cook the shrimp with all the sauce for about 3 minutes, until cooked through and opaque. Transfer to a clean bowl.

4. Place another large skillet over medium heat. Add the remaining 1 teaspoon sesame oil, the spinach, and mushrooms. Sauté for 3 to 5 minutes until the spinach is soft and most of the moisture has evaporated. Transfer to a clean bowl.

5. Wipe the skillet clean and place it over high heat. Add the canola oil and tilt the pan to coat the bottom. Carefully crack the eggs into the pan and fry for 3 to 5 minutes until set.

6. Evenly divide the cooked rice among 4 serving bowls. Top each with cooked shrimp and spinach, then finish with a fried egg.

7. Sprinkle with sesame seeds, and serve with kimchee (if using) and additional soy sauce.

Nutrition:

Calories: 586 Cal

Fat: 17g

Carbs: 67g

Fiber: 2g

Protein: 39g

41. Coconut-Crusted Shrimp

Preparation Time: 10 Minutes

Cooking Time: 5-7 Minutes

Servings: 4

Ingredients:

- ¼ cup Whole-Grain Gluten-Free Flour Blend (see here).
- 1½ cups unsweetened shredded coconut.
- 2 egg whites.
- ½ teaspoon sea salt.
- ¼ teaspoon garlic powder.
- 1½ pounds jumbo shrimp, peeled and butterflied.
- ¼ cup coconut oil.

Directions:

1. Place the flour blend in a small bowl.
2. Place the coconut in another small bowl.
3. In a third small bowl, whisk the egg whites, salt, and garlic powder.
4. Dip each shrimp into the flour blend, then the egg white mixture, and then dredge in the coconut. Place each on a plate.
5. Heat a large skillet or sauté pan over medium-high heat until hot, about 2 minutes.

6. Melt the coconut oil in the skillet and tilt the pan to coat the bottom.

7. When the oil is hot, transfer the shrimp to the pan and cook for 2 to 3 minutes on each side until golden brown, crisp, and cooked through.

Nutrition:

Calories: 383 Cal

Fat: 24g

Carbs: 11g

Fiber: 3g

Protein: 34g

42. Steamed Mussels

Preparation Time: 10 Minutes

Cooking Time: 15 Minutes

Servings: 4

Ingredients:

- 2 tablespoons extra-virgin olive oil.
- 3 tablespoons cold butter, divided.
- 1 yellow onion, diced.
- 4 garlic cloves, minced.
- 1 teaspoon fresh thyme leaves.
- 3 pounds fresh mussels, scrubbed and debearded.
- ½ cup dry white wine.
- Sea salt.
- Freshly ground black pepper.
- ½ cup roughly chopped fresh parsley.
- 1 lemon, halved.

Directions:

1. In a large pot over medium heat, heat the olive oil and melt 1 tablespoon of the butter.
2. Add the onion, garlic, and thyme and cook for about 5 minutes, until the onion is somewhat softened.

3. Add the mussels and white wine and give everything a good toss. Season generously with salt and pepper. Cover and cook until the mussels steam open, about 5 minutes.
4. Transfer any opened mussels to a serving dish, while cooking the rest until all are opened. Discard any mussels that have not opened after 10 minutes.
5. Continue simmering the pan juices for another 2 to 3 minutes until somewhat reduced.
6. Whisk in the remaining 2 tablespoons butter, one tablespoon at a time, to thicken the sauce. Pour the sauce over the mussels.
7. Shower with the fresh parsley and squeeze the lemon juice over, watching for any seeds. Serve immediately.

Nutrition:

Calories: 472 Cal

Fat: 23g

Carbs: 18g

Fiber: 1g

Protein: 41g

Chapter 7 Other Dinner Recipes

43. Seared Sea Scallops

Preparation Time: 2 Minutes

Cooking Time: 12-16 Minutes

Servings: 4

Ingredients:

- 2 tablespoons extra-virgin olive oil, divided.
- 2 tablespoons butter, divided.
- 1½ pounds jumbo or colossal sea scallops.
- Sea salt.
- Freshly ground black pepper.

Directions:

1. Heat a large skillet or sauté pan over medium-high heat until hot. Heat 1 tablespoon of the olive oil and melt 1 tablespoon of the butter in the skillet and swirl the pan to coat.

2. Pat half of the scallops dry with a paper towel. Season generously with salt and pepper.

3. When the butter foams and begins to brown, place the seasoned scallops into the pan. Cook for 2 to 3 minutes until a golden-brown crust forms on the bottom, basting continuously with the pan juices.

4. Flip the scallops and cook for 1 minute, basting as you go. Transfer the cooked scallops to a warmed serving dish.

5. Add the remaining 1 tablespoon olive oil and the butter to the skillet. Cook the remaining scallops as in steps 2 and 3. Transfer the cooked scallops to the serving dish and serve immediately.

Nutrition:

Calories: 261 Cal

Fat: 14g

Carbs: 4g

Fiber: 0g

Protein: 29g

44. Chile Lime Cod

Preparation Time: 5 Minutes

Cooking Time: 15 Minutes

Servings: 4

Ingredients:

- 4 (6-ounce) cod fillets.
- Juice of 1 lime.
- Zest of 1 lime.
- 1 tablespoon ancho chile powder.
- 1 teaspoon smoked paprika.
- 1 teaspoon ground coriander.
- ½ teaspoon sea salt.
- ¼ teaspoon freshly ground black pepper.
- ⅛ Teaspoon cayenne pepper.
- 2 tablespoons canola oil.

Directions:

1. Pat the cod fillets dry with a paper towel and put on a plate. Sprinkle each fillet evenly with the lime juice.
2. In a shallow dish, mix the lime zest, ancho chile powder, paprika, coriander, salt, black pepper, and cayenne pepper.
3. Coat the cod fillets with the spice mixture.
4. In a large skillet or sauté pan over medium-high heat, heat the canola oil until hot.

202

5. Sear the fish for 3 to 4 minutes on each side, or until cooked through and the fish flakes easily with a fork.

Nutrition:

Calories: 242 Cal

Fat: 9g

Carbs: 0g

Fiber: 0g

Protein: 39g

45. Pan-Seared Chicken Breast with Sautéed Zucchini

Preparation Time: 5 Minutes

Cooking Time: 20 Minutes

Servings: 4

Ingredients:

- 2 to 3 tablespoons extra-virgin olive oil, divided.
- 3 to 4 (4- to 6-ounce) boneless skinless chicken breasts, pounded to a uniform ½-inch thickness.
- Sea salt.
- Freshly ground black pepper.
- 2 medium zucchini, quartered lengthwise, cut into ½-inch pieces.
- ½ cup dry red wine, such as Merlot.

Directions:

1. Heat a large skillet or sauté pan over medium-high heat until hot, about 2 minutes. Add 1 tablespoon of the olive oil to the pan and tilt the pan to coat the bottom.

2. Pat the chicken breasts dry with paper towels and liberally season both sides with salt and pepper. Place in the skillet and cook for 5 minutes until well browned. Flip and cook for 4 to 5 minutes on the other side until cooked through. Transfer to serving plates.

204

3. Return the skillet to medium-high heat and add another 1 tablespoon olive oil to the pan.

4. Add the zucchini and sauté for about 3 minutes, until browned on the outside but still somewhat firm. Season with salt and pepper, and transfer to the serving plates.

5. Carefully add the red wine to the pan. Simmer for about 2 minutes, stirring frequently, until reduced to a few tablespoons.

6. Drizzle in 1 to 2 teaspoons of the remaining olive oil and whisk to combine. Pour the sauce over the chicken and zucchini and serve.

Nutrition:

Calories: 453Cal

Fat: 23g

Carbs: 4g

Fiber: 1g

Protein: 50g

46. Moroccan Chicken Tagine

Preparation Time: 15 Minutes

Cooking Time: 45 Minutes

Servings: 4-5

Ingredients:

- 1 whole chicken (3-4 lbs), cut into pieces.
- 2 large onions, chopped.
- 2-3 garlic cloves, finely chopped or pressed.
- ½ cup green or black olives.
- 1 preserved lemon, quartered and deseeded.
- 5 tbsp. olive oil.
- 1 tsp. grated ginger.
- 1 tsp. cumin.
- 1 tbsp. paprika.
- 1 tsp. black pepper.
- 1 tsp. turmeric.
- ½ tsp. salt.
- 1 bunch of fresh coriander.
- 1 bunch of fresh parsley.

Directions:

1. Rinse and dry chicken and place onto a clean plate.

2. In a large bowl, mix three tablespoons of olive oil, salt, half the onions, garlic, ginger, cumin, paprika, and turmeric. Mix thoroughly, crush the garlic with your fingers, and add a little water to make a paste.
3. Roll the chicken pieces into the marinade and leave for 10-15 minutes.
4. Heat a deep casserole with a lid and add 2 tablespoons of olive oil. Add the chicken and pour excess marinade juices over the top. Add the remaining onions, olives and chopped preserved lemon. Tie the parsley and coriander together into a bouquet and place it on top of the chicken.
5. Cover, bring to a boil and immediately reduce to a simmer. Cook for 45 minutes or until the chicken is cooked through and quite tender. Serve with rice or quinoa.

Nutrition:

Calories: 280 Cal

Fat: 8g

Carbs: 34g

Fiber: 6g

Protein: 19g

47. Mediterranean Chicken with Buckwheat

Preparation Time: 5 Minutes

Cooking Time: 15 Minutes

Servings: 4-5

Ingredients:

- 2 chicken breast halves, cut into strips.
- 2 garlic cloves, finely chopped.
- 1 cup chicken broth
- 1 lemon, rind finely grated, juiced.
- 1 cup buckwheat.
- 1 cup cherry tomatoes, halved.
- ½ cup green olives, pitted, halved.
- ½ cup fresh parsley leaves, chopped.
- 5-6 spring onions, trimmed, chopped.
- 2 tbsp. drained capers.
- 3 tbsp. olive oil.
- ½ tsp. freshly ground black pepper.

Directions:

1. Marinate the chicken in the oil, garlic and black pepper in a shallow dish. Heat an ovenproof casserole over medium-high heat.

2. Add half the chicken mixture and cook for 2-3 minutes, tossing, until just cooked.
3. Transfer to a plate, cover with foil to keep warm and set aside. Repeat with the remaining chicken mixture.
4. Heat a large, dry saucepan and toast the buckwheat for about three minutes.
5. Add the toasted buckwheat to the casserole together with broth and lemon juice.
6. Add in the chicken, lemon rind, tomatoes, olives, parsley, spring onions and capers.
7. Toss well to combine and bake in a preheated to 350°F for 15 minutes.

Nutrition:

Calories: 196 Cal

Fat: 3g

Carbs: 33g

Fiber: 7g

Protein: 13g

48. Chicken Moussaka

Preparation Time: 30 Minutes

Cooking Time: 40 Minutes

Servings: 6

Ingredients:

- 2 big eggplants cut into ½ inch thick rounds.
- Olive oil cooking spray.
- 1 tbsp. salt.
- 1 onion, finely cut.
- ½ tsp. cinnamon.
- ½ tsp. nutmeg.
- 1/4 tsp. coriander.
- 1/4 tsp. grated ginger.
- 2 cups canned tomatoes, undrained, chopped.
- 2 cups shredded roast chicken.
- ½ cup finely chopped fresh parsley leaves.
- 1 tsp. sugar.
- 1 cup yogurt.
- 1 cup Parmesan cheese.
- Salt and black pepper, to taste.

Directions:

1. Place eggplant slices on a tray and sprinkle with plenty of salt. Let sit for 30 minutes, then rinse with cold water. Lay slices out flat and use a clean kitchen towel to squeeze out excess water and pat dry.

2. Heat a frying pan over medium-high heat. Spray both sides of eggplant with oil. Cook in batches for3-4 minutes each side or until golden. Transfer to a plate.

3. In the same pan sauté onion, stirring, for 3-4 minutes or until softened. Add spice. Sauté for one minute until fragrant. Add tomatoes and sugar, stir, and sauté until thickened. Add chicken and parsley and stir well to combine.

4. Arrange half the eggplant slices in a baking dish. Cover with chicken and tomato mixture and arrange remaining eggplant. Top with yogurt and sprinkle with Parmesan cheese. Bake for 30 minutes or until golden. Set aside for five minutes and serve.

Nutrition:

Calories: 347 Cal

Fat: 5g

Carbs: 32g

Fiber: 6g

Protein: 45g

49. Chicken and Artichoke Rice

Preparation Time: 25 Minutes

Cooking Time: 25 Minutes

Servings: 4

Ingredients:

- 3 skinless chicken breasts, cut into strips.
- 2 leeks, white parts only, chopped.
- 4-5 chargrilled artichokes hearts, quartered.
- 2 garlic cloves, crushed.
- 1/3 cup rice.
- 1 cup chicken broth.
- 2 tbsp. olive oil.
- 1 tsp. lemon rind.
- 7-8 fresh basil leaves, chopped.
- 1 bay leaf.
- Juice of 1 lemon.

Directions:

1. Heat the oil in a large saucepan over low heat. Gently sauté the leeks, bay leaf and garlic for about 3-4 minutes, stirring occasionally. Add in the lemon rind and the chicken breasts and cook, stirring, for 5-6 minutes.

2. Add rice, stir, and add chicken broth and half the lemon juice. Bring to the boil, then reduce heat, cover, and cook for 10 minutes.
3. Set aside covered for 5 minutes then stir in the chopped basil, artichokes hearts and remaining lemon juice.

Nutrition:

Calories: 335 Cal

Fat: 17g

Carbs: 13g

Fiber: 1g

Protein: 31g

50. Easy Chicken Parmigiana

Preparation Time: 2 Minutes

Cooking Time: 20 Minutes

Servings: 4

Ingredients:

- 4 chicken breast fillets.
- 1 eggplant, peeled and sliced lengthwise.
- 1 can tomatoes, diced.
- 9 oz. mozzarella cheese, sliced.
- 2 tbsp. olive oil.

Directions:

1. Place chicken into an ovenproof casserole. Heat olive oil in a non-stick frying pan and cook eggplant in batches, for 1-2 minutes each side, or until golden.
2. Place eggplant over the chicken and add in tomatoes.
3. Top with mozzarella slices and bake, in a preheated to 350 F, for 20 minutes, or until the cheese is golden.

Nutrition:

Calories: 208 Cal,Fat: 6g

Carbs: 10gFiber: 1g

Protein: 27g

Chapter 8 Snacks Recipe

51. Basil and Minced Pork Fajita

Preparation Time: 40 Minutes

Cooking Time: 40 Minutes

Servings: 4

Ingredients:

- 1 pound minced pork.
- 2 whole organic eggs.
- 2 Handful of basil leaves.
- 1 large onion, finely chopped.
- 2 large tomatoes, chopped.
- 4 large corn tortillas.
- 1 teaspoon garlic paste.
- 1 teaspoon Cajun spice.
- 3 tablespoons olive oil.
- Salt to taste.

Directions:

1. Whisk eggs in a large bowl until frothy and keep aside.
2. Heat olive oil in a large non-stick pan over medium-high flame. Stir in the chopped onion and sauté until golden-brown. Add garlic paste to the pan and cook for few seconds, stirring continuously.

3. Now, add Cajun spice, minced pork, basil and salt to the pan. Cook until pork is cooked through and turn golden-brown.
4. Then, add whisked eggs to the pan and cook for 5 minutes or until eggs are done, stirring occasionally.
5. Once done, remove the pan from heat and keep aside.
6. Heat another pan over medium-high flame. Put a corn tortilla in the hot pan and cook both sides until golden. Repeat the same procedure with the remaining tortilla.
7. Once done, place a tortilla over the chopping board and put cooked pork at one.
8. Add some chopped. Roll the end of tortilla with cooked pork and tomatoes towards the other end.
9. Repeat the same procedure with remaining tortillas and Ingredients.
10. Transfer the prepared fajitas to a serving platter.
11. Serve!

Nutrition:

Calories: 322 Cal

Fat: 22g

Carbs: 11g

Fiber: 2g

Protein: 23g

52. Tortilla Pocket

Preparation Time: 10 Minutes

Cooking Time: 10 Minutes

Servings: 6

Ingredients:

- 6 small tortillas.
- ½ pound roasted chicken breast.
- 2 cups boiled green peas.
- ½ teaspoon thyme, ground.
- Olive oil spray for greasing.
- Salt and pepper to taste.

Directions:

1. Preheat the oven to 200°C. Lightly grease a baking tray with olive oil spray and keep aside.
2. Shred the roasted chicken breast with the help of a fork.
3. Combine shredded chicken, boiled green peas, thyme, salt and pepper in a bowl. Mix well and keep aside.
4. Place a tortilla over a chopping board and put 1/6 portion of prepared chicken mix in the center. To make a square pocket, bring an edge to the center and the other edge overlapping the first one, then the third one and at last the fourth. Seal the pocket by screwing a toothpick in the center. Make 5 more pockets using the same Method.

5. Once done, place the pockets in the prepared baking tray and spray some olive oil over them.

6. Now, bake for 10-15 minutes until the tortillas turn crisp and golden.

7. Once done, remove the tray from the oven and place it over a wire rack to cool down a bit for about 5 minutes.

8. Transfer the pockets to a serving platter.

9. Serve hot with mayonnaise or ketchup.

Nutrition:

Calories: 312 Cal

Fat: 17g

Carbs: 35g

Fiber: 6g

Protein: 8g

53. Crispy Honey Chili Pork Tenderloins

Preparation Time: 10 Minutes

Cooking Time: 10-15 Minutes

Servings: 4

Ingredients:

- 1 pound pork tenderloins, diced into pieces (2x2 inches).
- 2 whole organic eggs.
- 4 tablespoons corn-flour.
- 2 tablespoons ginger-garlic paste.
- 2 tablespoons gluten-free soya sauce.
- ½ cup honey.
- 2 teaspoon chili flakes.
- Pomace olive oil for deep frying.
- Salt and pepper to taste.

Directions:

1. Combine eggs, corn-flour, ginger-garlic paste, gluten-free soya sauce, salt and pepper in a large bowl. Mix well until uniformly combined.

2. Now, add in diced tenderloins and mix well with hands until each piece is evenly coated with the prepared mix. Keep aside.

3. Heat pomace olive oil in a deep bottom pan over medium-high flame. Put battered tenderloin pieces in the pan with hot oil (one by one) and fry until golden-brown.

4. Once done, remove the tenderloin pieces from pan with the help of a strainer and place them over a paper towel so that it can absorb the extra oil. Keep aside.

5. Combine honey and chili flakes in a large bowl. Put fried tenderloin pieces in it. Mix well until all the pieces are evenly coated honey-chili mix.

6. Then, transfer the prepared dish to a serving platter.

7. Serve hot!

Nutrition:

Calories: 428 Cal

Fat: 22g

Carbs: 9g

Fiber: 0g

Protein: 47 g

54. Chicken and Potato Taco

Preparation Time: 30 Minutes

Cooking Time: 40 Minutes

Servings: 6

Ingredients:

- 1 pound chicken, boneless and skinless.
- 2 large potatoes, chopped into bite size pieces.
- 6 medium corn tortillas.
- Rings of 2 small large onions.
- 1 head of lettuce, finely chopped.
- 1 cucumber, thinly sliced.
- Handful of parsley leaves, finely chopped.
- 1 teaspoon garlic powder.
- 3 tablespoons peanut oil.
- Salt and pepper to taste.

Directions:

1. Cut the chicken into bite-size pieces and set aside.
2. Heat peanut oil in a large nonstick pan over medium-high heat. Add chopped potatoes and chicken pieces to the pan. Add in garlic powder, salt and pepper. Mix well and cover the pan with a lid. Let it simmer over low heat until chicken and potatoes are cooked through, stirring occasionally.

222

3. Once done, remove the pan from heat and keep aside.

4. Heat a pan over a medium-high flame and put a tortilla in it. Cook both sides until golden. Repeat the same procedure with remaining tortillas.

5. Now, place a warm corn tortilla over the chopping board. Put some cooked chicken and potatoes in the center. Put some finely chopped lettuce, onion rings, thinly sliced cucumber, finely chopped fresh parsley leaves on the top of cooked chicken-potatoes. Fold the tortilla into half and put it in the serving platter.

6. Repeat the same procedure with remaining Ingredients.

7. Serve warm.

Nutrition:

Calories: 396 Cal

Fat: 13g

Carbs: 45g

Fiber: 7g

Protein: 25g

55. Mexican Cheese Poblanos

Preparation Time: 10 Minutes

Cooking Time: 10 Minutes

Servings: 8

Ingredients:

- 8 poblano chilies.
- 12 tablespoons Philadelphia cream cheese.
- 4 whole organic eggs.
- 3 tablespoons corn flour.
- 3 tablespoon gluten-free breadcrumbs.
- Pomace olive oil for deep frying.
- Salt and pepper to taste.

Directions:

1. Make a vertical slit in each chili and remove the seeds from them. Keep aside.
2. Whisk eggs in a large bowl until frothy. Add in cornflour, gluten-free breadcrumbs, salt and pepper. Mix well and keep aside.
3. Heat olive oil in a deep bottom pan over medium-high flame. Stuff each pepper with 1 ½ tablespoon of cream cheese.

4. Then, evenly coated the stuffed peppers with prepared egg mix and put them in the pan with hot (one by one). Fry until golden-crisp.
5. Once done, remove the peppers from the pan with the help of a strainer and place them over a paper towel so that it can absorb the extra oil.
6. Now, transfer the fried pepper to a serving platter.
7. Serve hot with Mexican chili.

Nutrition:

Calories: 259 Cal

Fat: 17g

Carbs: 17 g

Fiber: 3g

Protein: 13g

56. Three Cheese Nachos

Preparation Time: 20 Minutes

Cooking Time: 10 Minutes

Servings: 2

Ingredients:

- 4 medium corn tortillas.
- 1 cup mozzarella cheese.
- ½ cup parmesan cheese.
- ½ cup cheddar cheese.
- 1 cup jalapeno slices.
- 1 large onion, finely chopped.
- 1 large tomato, finely chopped.
- Pomace olive oil for deep frying.

Directions:

1. Make 8 nachos out of each tortilla with the help of a knife.
2. Heat pomace olive oil in a deep bottom pan over medium-high flame. Put nachos in the pan with hot oil (one by one). Fry until golden and crisp.
3. Once done, remove the nachos from the pan with the help of a strainer and place them over a paper towel so that it can absorb the extra oil. Keep aside and let them come to room temperature.
4. Combine all the cheese in a bowl and keep aside.

5. Now place the fried nachos in microwave-safe dish in a single layer. Sprinkle three cheese on the top and put jalapeno slices over it.

6. Microwave for 1-2 minutes or until cheese melts down completely.

7. Once done, remove cheese nachos from the microwave. 8. Top with chopped onion and tomatoes.

Nutrition:

Calories: 153 Cal

Fat: 4g

Carbs: 21g

Fiber: 3g

Protein: 9g

57. Butter Cajun Shrimps

Preparation Time: 5 Minutes

Cooking Time: 10 Minutes

Servings: 2

Ingredients:

- ½ pound shrimps, deveined and peeled.
- 1 teaspoon Cajun spice.
- 3 tablespoons butter.
- Salt and pepper to taste.

Directions:

1. Melt butter in a large and deep bottom pot over medium-high heat. Add all the ingredients to the pan. Cook until shrimps turn pink and translucent, stirring occasionally.
2. Once done, remove the pan from heat and transfer the shrimps to a serving platter.

Nutrition:

Calories: 362 Cal

Fat: 21g

Carbs: 28g

Fiber: 3g

Protein: 18g

58. Smokey Chili Lamb Bites

Preparation Time: 10 Minutes

Cooking Time: 1 Hour

Servings: 2

Ingredients:

- ½ pound lamb, boneless and diced into bite-size pieces.
- 1 tablespoon hot sauce.
- 2 teaspoons garlic paste.
- 1 teaspoon roasted cumin powder.
- 3 drops of liquid smoke.
- 2 tablespoon pomace olive oil.
- Salt to taste.

Directions:

1. Put all the ingredients in a large bowl and mix well. Keep aside.
2. Heat olive oil in a large non-stick pan over medium-high flame. Put lamb bites in the pan and pour in 1 quart of water.
3. Cover the pan with the lid. Let it simmer over low heat until the lamb is cooked through and water evaporates completely, about an hour.

4. Once done, remove the pan from heat and transfer the lamb bites to a serving platter.
5. Serve hot!

Nutrition:

Calories: 289 Cal

Fat: 10g

Carbs: 33g

Fiber: 10g Protein: 20g

59. Jalapeno Yogurt Balls

Preparation Time: 15 Minutes

Cooking Time: 5 Minutes

Servings: 10

Ingredients:

- 1 cup Greek yogurt.
- 3 cups gluten-free bread crumbs.
- ½ cup jalapenos, finely chopped.
- Pomace olive oil for deep frying.
- Salt and pepper to taste.

Directions:

1. Combine Greek yogurt, bread crumbs, jalapeno, salt and pepper in a large bowl. Mix well and make 10 balls using your hands. Keep aside.
2. Heat olive oil in a deep bottom pan over medium-high flame. Put prepared balls into the pan and fry until golden-brown.
3. Once done, take out the balls from the pan with the help of a strainer and place them over a paper towel so that it can absorb the extra oil.
4. Transfer the balls to a serving platter. 5. Serve hot with ketchup!

Nutrition:

Calories: 28 Cal

Fat: 0g

Carbs: 2g

Fiber: 0g

Protein: 5g

60. Potato and Green Pea Cutlets

Preparation Time: 10 Minutes

Cooking Time: 5 Minutes

Servings: 8

Ingredients:

- 2 large potatoes, boiled and peeled.
- 1 medium onion, finely chopped.
- ½ cup boiled green peas.
- ½ teaspoon cumin seeds.
- Pomace olive oil for shallow frying.
- Salt and pepper to taste.

Directions:

1. Mash boiled potatoes in a large bowl with a fork until smooth. Add in onion, green peas, cumin seeds, salt and pepper. Mix well and make 8 cutlets using your hands. Keep aside.
2. Heat olive oil in a deep bottom pan over medium-high flame. Put prepared cutlets into the pan and fry until golden-brown.
3. Once done, take out the cutlets from the pan with the help of a strainer and place them over a paper towel so that it can absorb the extra oil.
4. Transfer the cutlets to a serving platter.
5. Serve hot with ketchup!

Nutrition:

Calories: 117 Cal

Fat: 0g

Carbs: 24g

Fiber: 4g Protein: 4g

Chapter 9 Other Snack Recipes

61. Avocado Crust California Pizza

Preparation Time: 30 Minutes

Cooking Time: 15 Minutes

Servings: 2

Ingredients:

- 1 cup potato starch or tapioca flour, plus more for sprinkling.
- 2 large avocados, peeled and pitted, divided.
- ½ teaspoon freshly squeezed lemon juice.
- ½ teaspoon baking powder.
- ⅛ Teaspoon salt.
- 2 to 3 tablespoons water.
- ¾ cup shredded vegan mozzarella cheese.
- 1 Roma tomato, sliced.
- 1 Yukon Gold potato, baked until tender and diced.
- 2 garlic cloves, minced.
- 1 small shallot, thinly sliced.
- Store-bought vegan pesto (optional).
- 1 to 2 tablespoons extra-virgin olive oil.
- Kosher salt.
- Freshly ground black pepper.

Directions:

1. Preheat the oven to 500°F. Sprinkle a piece of parchment paper with potato starch. Place a pizza stone or baking sheet in the oven to heat for 30 minutes.
2. In a food processor, combine one of the avocados, the potato starch, lemon juice, baking powder, and salt. Blend until smooth. Slowly add 2 tablespoons of water until it forms dough. Add 1 more tablespoon of water if needed. The dough should be pliable and soft, but not overly sticky.
3. Place the dough on the prepared parchment. Using your hands, press the dough to form a ¼-inch-thick, 12-inch-round disk. Top the dough evenly with the cheese, tomato, potato, garlic, and shallot. Drizzle with the pesto (if using) and oil.
4. Carefully transfer the parchment paper with the dough to the heated pizza stone. Bake until the cheese is golden and bubbly, about 15 minutes.
5. Meanwhile, cube the remaining avocado. Let the pizza cool for 5 minutes, top with the avocado, season with salt and pepper to taste, slice, and serve.

Nutrition:

Calories: 178 Cal

Fat: 12g,Carbs: 16g,Fiber: 5g

Protein: 4g

62. Cauliflower Crust Margarita Pizza

Preparation Time: 30 Minutes

Cooking Time: 30 Minutes

Servings: 4

Ingredients:

- 1 head cauliflower, chopped.
- ¼ cup water.
- 1 tablespoon arrowroot.
- 1 tablespoon extra-virgin olive oil or avocado oil.
- 1 tablespoon baking powder.
- ⅔ Cup potato starch.
- 1 teaspoon salt, plus more as needed.
- 1 cup shredded vegan mozzarella cheese.
- 1 Roma tomato, sliced.
- Fresh basil leaves, for garnish.
- Freshly ground black pepper.

Directions:

1. Preheat the oven to 500°F. Place a pizza stone or baking sheet in the oven and heat for 30 minutes. Flour a piece of parchment paper.

2. Put the cauliflower in a food processor, and process on high until finely chopped and the consistency of rice. Transfer to a medium glass bowl. Microwave on high until tender, 2 to 3 minutes. Let cool until able to handle.

3. Meanwhile, in a small bowl, whisk together the water, arrowroot, oil, and baking powder.

4. Place a nut bag or large dish towel over a large empty bowl. Add the cauliflower rice and squeeze the bag around the cauliflower; water should drain into the bowl. Continue squeezing until the water is removed.

5. In a separate large bowl, combine the cauliflower rice, potato starch, salt, and arrowroot mixture. Stir until a dough forms. If the dough seems too dry to shape, add more water, 1 teaspoon at a time.

6. Place the dough on the prepared parchment. Roll the dough to form a ¼-inch-thick, 12-inch-round disk. Carefully transfer the parchment paper with the dough to the heated pizza stone. Bake for 10 minutes, then carefully flip the crust and bake until lightly golden, about 10 minutes.

7. Top the pizza evenly with the cheese and tomato. Bake until the cheese melts, 5 to 7 minutes. Remove from the

oven, garnish with basil, season with salt and pepper to taste, slice, and serve.

Nutrition:

Calories: 60 Cal

Fat: 3g

Carbs: 4g

Fiber: 1g

Protein: 4g

63. Sweet Potato-Crusted Pizza with Sun-Dried Tomato Pesto, Portobello, and Grilled Chicken

Preparation Time: 25 Minutes

Cooking Time: 20 Minutes

Servings: 2

Ingredients:

For the sun-dried tomato pesto.

- 4 ounces fresh basil leaves (about 2 handfuls).
- 4 ounces sun-dried tomatoes in olive oil.
- ¼ cup extra-virgin olive oil.
- ¼ cup chopped walnuts.
- 1 tablespoon freshly squeezed lemon juice.
- 1 teaspoon apple cider vinegar.
- ½ teaspoon salt.
- 1 garlic clove, minced.
- For the sweet potato crust.
- 1 large sweet potato, baked, peeled, and mashed (about 2 cups; see prep tip).
- 1 cup potato starch of cornstarch, plus extra for sprinkling.
- ½ teaspoon freshly squeezed lemon juice.
- 1 teaspoon baking powder.

- ⅛ Teaspoon salt.

For the toppings.

- 1 cup diced grilled chicken.
- ½ cup shredded vegan mozzarella cheese.
- 1 Portobello mushroom, stemmed and diced.
- 2 tablespoons chopped walnuts.

Directions:

1. For the pesto, in a food processor, put the basil, sun-dried tomatoes, oil, walnuts, lemon juice, vinegar, salt, and garlic. Blend on high until smooth. Pour into a small bowl.
2. For the sweet potato crust, preheat the oven to 500°F. Place a pizza stone or baking sheet in the oven to heat for 30 minutes. Sprinkle a piece of parchment paper with potato starch.
3. Wash and dry the food processor bowl. Put the sweet potato, potato starch, lemon juice, baking powder, and salt in the food processor. Pulse until a dough forms.
4. Place the dough on the prepared parchment. Using your hands, press the dough to form a ¼-inch-thick, 12-inch-round disk. Bake for 20 minutes. Lightly spread the pesto over the crust, leaving 1 inch uncovered around the edge.

5. For the toppings, sprinkle the chicken, cheese, mushroom, and walnuts over the pesto in the order listed. Bake until slightly browned and most of the liquid from the vegetables evaporates, 10 to 15 minutes.
6. Let cool for 5 minutes, season with salt and pepper to taste, slice, and serve.

Nutrition:

Calories: 169 Cal

Fat: 0g

Carbs: 38g

Fiber: 3g

Protein: 4g

64. Flatbread

Preparation Time: 15 Minutes

Cooking Time: 25 Minutes

Servings: 4

Ingredients:

- 1¼ cup plain dairy-free yogurt.
- 2 tablespoons plus 4 teaspoons extra-virgin olive oil, divided.
- 1 teaspoon apple cider vinegar.
- 2 cups Basic Gluten-Free Flour Blend or store-bought equivalent.
- ¼ cup tapioca flour.
- 1 tablespoon baking powder.
- 1 teaspoon salt.
- ¼ teaspoon baking soda.

Directions:

1. In a large bowl, whisk together the yogurt, 2 tablespoons of oil, and the vinegar. Add the flour blend, tapioca flour, baking powder, salt, and baking soda. With a spatula, stir together until a dough forms. Knead with your hands or the spatula for 3 minutes.

2. Divide the dough into four disks. On a floured work surface, place one of the disks and, using a rolling pin, roll

to a ¼-inch thickness. Repeat with the remaining dough disks.

3. In a large nonstick skillet over medium-high heat, heat 1 teaspoon of oil. Add one dough disk to the skillet and cook until slightly browned and crisp, 2 to 3 minutes per side. Transfer to a platter and repeat with the remaining dough, adding 1 teaspoon of oil to the pan for each piece of dough.

Nutrition:

Calories: 85 Cal

Fat: 1g

Carbs: 16g

Fiber: 3g

Protein: 5g

65. Garlic Butter Flatbread Sticks

Preparation Time: 15 Minutes

Cooking Time: 10 Minutes

Servings: 16

Ingredients:

- 1 recipe Flatbread.
- 4 tablespoons vegan butter, melted.
- 8 garlic cloves, minced.
- Kosher salt.
- Freshly ground black pepper.

Directions:

1. Preheat the oven to 400°F. Line a large baking sheet with parchment paper or a silicone baking mat.
2. In a small glass bowl, microwave the butter until melted, about 30 seconds. Stir in the garlic. Place the flatbread on the prepared baking sheet. With a basting brush, brush them with the garlic butter. Season with salt and pepper to taste. Cut each flatbread into four strips.
3. Bake until crispy, 5 to 10 minutes.

Nutrition:

Calories: 102 Cal

Fat: 2g

Carbs: 19g

Fiber: 1g

Protein: 3g

66. Graham Crackers

Preparation Time: 35 Minutes

Cooking Time: 15 Minutes

Servings: 20 Crackers

Ingredients:

- 1½ cups brown rice flour, plus more for sprinkling.
- ½ cup potato starch.
- ⅓ Cup packed light brown sugar or coconut sugar.
- 6 tablespoons unsweetened dairy-free milk.
- 5 tablespoons vegan butter.
- 3 tablespoons honey.
- 1 teaspoon baking powder.
- ½ teaspoon salt.
- 1 teaspoon molasses.
- 1 teaspoon granulated sugar (optional).

Directions:

1. Preheat the oven to 350°F. Lightly flour two pieces of parchment paper.

2. In a food processor, combine the flour, potato starch, sugar, milk, butter, honey, baking powder, salt, and molasses. Pulse until combined. Do not over mix or it will become warm and sticky. If the dough is dry and crumbly, add more milk, 1 teaspoon at a time, until a stiff dough forms.

3. Divide the dough in half and place one piece on one of the prepared pieces of parchment. Pat to form a rectangular shape. Sprinkle the top lightly with more flour and place another piece of parchment paper on top. Roll the dough to a ⅛-inch thickness. Try to keep the dough the same thickness, especially at the edges, to avoid burning. Using a pizza cutter, cut the dough into 2-by-3½-inch rectangles. No need to separate the slices as they will break apart after baking. Repeat this process with the remaining dough.

4. Transfer the dough, on the parchment sheets, to two small baking sheets and place in the freezer for 10 minutes.

5. Remove from the freezer and pierce the tops with several holes using the end of an ice pop stick or fork. This helps make the crackers crisp. Lightly sprinkle the tops with the granulated sugar (if using).

6. Bake until lightly golden, about 15 minutes. Let cool for 10 minutes, then transfer on the parchment to a wire rack to cool completely.

Nutrition:

Calories: 93 Cal

Fat: 0g

Carbs: 22g

Fiber: 1g

Protein: 2g

67. Gluten-Free Crackers

Preparation Time: 35 Minutes

Cooking Time: 15 Minutes

Servings: 44 Crackers

Ingredients:

- 1½ cups brown rice flour, plus more for sprinkling.
- ½ cup potato starch.
- 4 tablespoons vegan butter.
- 6 tablespoons water.
- 1 tablespoon maple syrup.
- ¾ teaspoon salt.
- ½ teaspoon baking powder.
- Kosher salt.

Directions:

1. Preheat the oven to 400°F. Lightly flour two pieces of parchment paper.
2. In a food processor, combine the flour, potato starch, butter, water, maple syrup, salt, and baking powder. Pulse until combined. Do not over mix or it will become warm and sticky. If the dough is dry and crumbly, add more water, 1 teaspoon at a time, until a stiff dough forms.
3. Divide the dough in half and place one piece on one of the prepared pieces of parchment. Pat to form a rectangular

shape. Sprinkle the top lightly with more flour and place another piece of parchment on top. Roll the dough to a ⅛-inch thickness. Try to keep the dough the same thickness, especially at the edges, to avoid burning. Using a pizza cutter, cut the dough into 2-by-3½-inch rectangles. No need to separate the slices as they will break apart after baking. Repeat this process with the second half of the dough.

4. Transfer the dough, on the parchment paper, to two small baking sheets, and place in the freezer for 10 minutes.

5. Remove from the freezer and pierce the top of each rectangle several times with a fork to create holes (like you see on butter crackers). This helps make the crackers crisp. Sprinkle the tops lightly with kosher salt.

6. Bake until slightly browned, about 15 minutes. Let cool for 10 minutes, then transfer on the parchment to a wire rack to cool completely.

Nutrition:

Calories: 163 Cal

Fat: 3g

Carbs: 30g

Fiber: 2g

Protein: 3g

Chapter 10 Extra Side Recipes

68. Cream of Chicken Soup

Preparation Time: 5 Minutes

Cooking Time: 15 Minutes

Servings: 4

Ingredients:

- 2 tablespoons unsalted butter.
- ½ cup all-purpose gluten-free flour blend.
- 2½ cups gluten-free chicken broth.
- 1¼ cups whole milk.
- 1 teaspoon salt.
- ½ teaspoon freshly ground black pepper.
- ½ teaspoon onion powder.
- ½ teaspoon garlic powder.
- ¼ teaspoon dried parsley.

Directions:

1. In a large saucepan, melt the butter over medium heat, then whisk in the flour blend.
2. Slowly whisk in the chicken broth, milk, salt, pepper, onion powder, garlic powder, and dried parsley. Whisking constantly, bring to a low boil.

3. Turn the heat down to low and stir constantly for 5 to 10 minutes, or until the mixture begins to thicken.

4. Remove from the heat. The soup will thicken more than it cools.

Nutrition:

Calories: 233 Cal

Fat: 14g

Carbs: 19g

Fiber: 2g

Protein: 10g

69. Caldo de Pollo

Preparation Time: 10 Minutes

Cooking Time: 2 Hours

Servings: 8

Ingredients:

- 10 cups water.
- 3 cups gluten-free chicken broth.
- 2 tablespoon minced garlic.
- 2 large boneless, skinless chicken breasts.
- 7 red potatoes, roughly chopped.
- 1 medium onion, roughly chopped.
- 2 cups baby carrots.
- 10 cabbage leaves, roughly chopped.
- 1 (28-ounce) can diced tomatoes.
- Pinch salt.
- Pinch freshly ground black pepper.
- 1 lemon, cut into 8 wedges (optional).

Directions:

1. In a large stockpot, combine the water, chicken broth, and garlic. Bring to a boil over medium-high heat.
2. Add the chicken breasts and reduce the heat to medium-low. Cook for 45 minutes.

3. Add the potatoes, onion, baby carrots, cabbage leaves, and tomatoes with their juice, salt, and pepper.

4. Cover the pot and cook for another 45 minutes, or until the veggies are soft and the chicken is cooked through. The chicken will be starting to fall apart; you can shred it with a fork if you like.

5. If desired, squeeze the fresh lemon juice into each bowl of soup just before serving.

Nutrition:

Calories: 298 Cal

Fat: 2g

Carbs: 40g

Fiber: 6g

Protein: 32g

70. Potato-Broccoli Soup

Preparation Time: 15 Minutes

Cooking Time: 30 Minutes

Servings: 4

Ingredients:

- 2 tablespoons unsalted butter.
- 1 small onion, finely chopped.
- 6 cups chopped broccoli florets.
- 2 large russet potatoes, peeled and diced.
- 1 tablespoon minced garlic.
- 2 cups gluten-free vegetable broth.
- 2 cups whole milk.
- ¼ teaspoon ground nutmeg (optional).
- Pinch salt.
- Pinch freshly ground black pepper

Directions:

1. In a large saucepan, melt the butter over medium heat. Add the onion and sauté for 2 to 3 minutes, or until soft.
2. Add the broccoli, potatoes, and garlic. Cover and cook for 5 minutes.
3. Add the vegetable broth and bring to a boil, then turn the heat back down to a simmer for 15 minutes, or until the vegetables are tender when pierced with a fork.

4. With an immersion blender, purée the vegetables until completely smooth or still a little chunky, depending on your preference.
5. Stir in the milk, nutmeg (if using), salt, and pepper.
6. Gently heat the soup over low heat for 5 to 8 minutes, or until heated through.

Nutrition:

Calories: 314 Cal

Fat: 10g

Carbs: 48g

Fiber: 8g

Protein: 11g

71. Cream of Mushroom Soup

Preparation Time: 5 Minutes

Cooking Time: 20 Minutes

Servings: 4

Ingredients:

- 4 tablespoons (½ stick) unsalted butter.
- 12 ounces white mushrooms, finely chopped.
- ¼ cup all-purpose gluten-free flour blend.
- 2 cups gluten-free chicken broth.
- 1⅓ cups whole milk.
- 1 tablespoon freshly squeezed lemon juice.
- 1 tablespoon dried parsley.
- Pinch salt.
- Pinch freshly ground black pepper.

Directions:

1. In a large saucepan, melt the butter over medium heat. Add the mushrooms and gently cook for 5 minutes.
2. Stir in the flour blend, then gradually add the broth.
3. Bring to a boil, then reduce the heat and simmer for 10 minutes.
4. Stir in the milk, lemon juice, parsley, salt, and pepper.
5. Gently heat the soup over low heat for 5 to 8 minutes, or until heated through. Serve immediately.

Nutrition:

Calories: 294 Cal

Fat: 19g

Carbs: 20g Fiber: 2g Protein: 13g

72. Strawberry-Cucumber Salad

Preparation Time: 10 Minutes

Cooking Time: 0 Minutes

Servings: 4

Ingredients:

- 2 large cucumbers, sliced.
- 2 cups sliced strawberries.
- ½ medium onion, sliced.
- ¼ cup balsamic vinegar.
- 2 tablespoons mild olive oil.
- ½ cup feta cheese.

Directions:

1. In a large bowl, toss together the cucumbers, strawberries, onion, balsamic vinegar, and olive oil.
2. Top with feta cheese before serving.

Nutrition:

Calories: 164 Cal

Fat: 11g

Carbs: 13g

Fiber: 3g

Protein: 4g

73. Mason Jar Taco Salad

Preparation Time: 15 Minutes

Cooking Time: 15 Minutes

Servings: 5

Ingredients:

- 1 pound lean ground beef.
- ¼ cup Homemade Taco Seasoning (here).
- ¼ cup water.
- 1½ cups gluten-free salsa.
- 5 tablespoons sour cream.
- 1-quart cherry tomatoes, chopped.
- 1 small onion, chopped.
- 2 avocados, halved, pitted, peeled, and chopped.
- Juice of ½ lime.
- 5 cups chopped romaine lettuce.

Directions:

1. In a medium pan, cook the ground beef over medium heat for 7 to 10 minutes, or until it's no longer pink. Drain off the grease.
2. Add the taco seasoning and water, and cook until most of the water evaporates. Allow the taco mixture to cool.
3. Divide the ingredients among 5 wide-mouths, 1-quart mason jars so that each contains the following layers in the following order: salsa, sour cream, tomatoes, onion, avocados, lime juice, taco mixture, and lettuce.
4. Seal the jars and store in the refrigerator for up to 5 days.
5. When you're ready to eat, place the contents into a bowl— or just grab a fork and eat straight from the jar.

Nutrition:

Calories: 512 Cal

Fat: 26g

Carbs: 40g

Fiber: 14g

Protein: 37g

74. Lemony Kale Salad with Parmesan and Golden Raisins

Preparation Time: 5 Minutes + 1 Hour to chill

Cooking Time: 0 Minutes

Servings: 4

Ingredients:

- 6 cups chopped curly kale.
- ¼ cup olive oil.
- Juice of 1 lemon.
- ½ cup grated Parmesan cheese.
- ½ cup golden raisins.

Directions:

1. In a large bowl, toss the kale with the olive oil and lemon juice.
2. Mix in the Parmesan cheese and golden raisins.
3. Refrigerate until chilled, about 1 hour.

Nutrition:

Calories: 257 Cal

Fat: 16g

Carbs: 25g, Fiber: 2g

Protein: 8g

75. Easy Three-Bean Salad

Preparation Time: 15 Minutes + 3 Hours to chill

Cooking Time: 0 Minute

Servings: 8

Ingredients:

- 1 (15-ounce) can black beans, drained and rinsed.
- 1 (15-ounce) can red kidney beans, drained and rinsed.
- 1 (15-ounce) can chickpeas, drained and rinsed.
- ½ medium red onion, finely chopped.
- ½ cup apple cider vinegar.
- ¼ cup honey.
- 3 tablespoons olive oil.
- 3 tablespoons dried parsley.
- 1 teaspoon salt.
- ½ teaspoons freshly ground black pepper.

Directions:

1. In a large bowl, toss together the black beans, kidney beans, chickpeas, and onion.
2. In a small bowl, whisk together the vinegar, honey, olive oil, parsley, salt, and pepper.
3. Pour the dressing over the beans and stir to coat. Cover and chill in the refrigerator for at least 3 hours or overnight.

Nutrition:

Calories: 266 Cal

Fat: 6g

Carbs: 43g

Fiber: 10g Protein: 10g

76. Mustard Potato Salad

Preparation Time: 15 Minutes + 4 Hours to chill

Cooking Time: 10 Minute

Servings: 4

Ingredients:

- 9 medium red potatoes, quartered.
- 2½ cups chopped broccoli florets.
- 1 small onion, chopped.
- ½ cup gluten-free.
- Dijon mustard.
- 2 teaspoons olive oil.
- 1 teaspoon gluten-free distilled white vinegar.
- Pinch salt.
- Pinch freshly ground black pepper.

Directions:

1. Fill a large pot with water and bring to a boil over high heat. Reduce the heat to low and add the potatoes and broccoli. Cook for 7 to 10 minutes, or until the potatoes are tender.
2. Drain the potatoes and broccoli in a colander and cool under cold running water.
3. In a large bowl, toss the cooled potatoes and broccoli with the onion.
4. In a small bowl, whisk together the mustard, olive oil, vinegar, salt, and pepper.
5. Pour the dressing over the potatoes and toss to coat.
6. Cover and chill in the refrigerator for at least 4 hours before serving.

Nutrition:

Calories: 266 Cal

Fat: 6g

Carbs: 43g

Fiber: 10g

Protein: 10g

Conclusion

The Gluten-free diet is genuinely life-changing. The diet improves your overall health and helps you lose the extra weight in a matter of days. The diet will show its multiple benefits even from the beginning, and it will become your new lifestyle soon.

As soon as you embrace this diet, you will start to live a completely new life. On the other hand, it is such a healthy option for your limited choices of food.

The collection we bring to you today is a combination of Gluten-free and vegetarian diets. You get to discover some fantastic Gluten-free, vegetarian dishes you can prepare in the comfort of your own home. All the recipes you found here follow both the rules, they all taste delicious and vibrant, and they are all easy to make.

Living gluten-free can be overwhelming when it comes to food preparation. Using your slow cooker makes it so much easier. You get great tasting food, one-pot meal, and easy cleanup!

So there you have it, the simplest way to live gluten-free with these easy to prepare and stress-free one-pot meals your family will love. I hope you found several to add to your go-to recipes.

This e-book can save you with the hassle of doing a month-long meal prepping with its delicious and simple recipes. The recipes are pretty simple and easy to stick to your gluten-free diet. And they deliver overall fantastic health benefits. You can even swap ingredients with your favorite ones and experiment with the recipes to make your meal plan that you will look forward to eating all month long.

Through this book, you have learned what gluten is, why it may be not right for you, and what it does to your body if you are sensitive to it. You have also learned how important it is to start the Gluten-Free Diet as soon as you have found out that you have gluten sensitivity or intolerance. This has also shown you the steps to take to get started on the Gluten-Free Diet and which foods you should choose and which to avoid. You have also acquired a variety of breakfast, main dish, and side dish recipes that will help you get started on the diet.

Now, you only have to collect more recipes and build healthy habits that will help you follow the Gluten-Free Diet easily, sustainably, and enjoyably. It may be not easy at times, but never give up on your health! All efforts are worth it when you have a body that is strong, healthy, and full of energy. It is, after all, the most priceless asset you have.

Most importantly, we hope you now see that living a gluten-free lifestyle is not impossible. It might not be one of the most natural things you will ever do, but it will enrich your life and your health far beyond anything you might ever have imagined.

We can assure you that such a combo is hard to find. So, start a gluten-free diet with a vegetarian "touch" today. It will be both useful and fun!

So, what are you still waiting for? Get with this diet and learn how to prepare the best and most flavored dishes. Enjoy them all!

Lightning Source UK Ltd.
Milton Keynes UK
UKHW020638151220
375092UK00003B/270